Bernd-Dietrich Katthagen

Bone Regeneration with Bone Substitutes

An Animal Study

With 101 Figures and 15 Tables

Springer-Verlag
Berlin Heidelberg New York
London Paris Tokyo

Priv.-Doz. Dr. med. Bernd-Dietrich Katthagen
Orthopädische Universitätsklinik und Poliklinik
Fachbereich 4, Klinische Medizin
D-6650 Homburg/Saar
Federal Republic of Germany

Title of the original German edition:
Hefte zur Unfallheilkunde, Heft 178
Knochenregeneration mit Knochenersatzmaterialien
© Springer-Verlag Berlin Heidelberg 1986
ISBN-13: 978-3-540-17425-7

ISBN-13: 978-3-540-17425-7 e-ISBN-13: 978-3-642-71827-4
DOI: 10.1007/978-3-642-71827-4

Library of Congress Cataloging-in-Publication Data. Katthagen, Bernd-Dietrich, 1952-. Bone regeneration with bone substitutes. Translation of: Knochenregeneration mit Knochenersatzmaterialien. Bibliography: p. Includes index. 1. Bone regeneration. 2. Bone-grafting. 3. Biomedical materials. I. Title.
RD123.K3813 1987 617'.471 87-4949
ISBN-13: 978-3-540-17425-7 (U.S.)

2124/3140-543210

Dedicated with gratitude
to my family

Acknowledgements

First of all, I wish to express my gratitude to my respected teacher, Professor H. Mittelmeier, for suggesting the present studies and for the valuable scientific advice and strong support which he has given me. I also wish to thank Professor G. Harbauer and Mrs. U. Diwo as well as the other co-workers of the Institute of Experimental Surgery of the University of Homburg for their effective support.

I am grateful to Mrs. U. Bechtel for the careful and rapid preparation of the histological sections; her interest in improving the histological technique deserves special mention. I wish to thank Professor V. Freitag for allowing me to use the microradiographical installations and Mrs. H. Konzmann for preparing the microradiographs. Professor R. Grillmaier introduced me to the histomorphometric technique for evaluation of histological sections. I wish to thank him for his kind support. I also wish to thank Professor R. Bock for the advice he gave me regarding the histomorphometric evaluation technique.

I am grateful to Kontron in Düsseldorf for letting me use the interactive picture analysis system (IBAS) for the histomorphometric investigations, to Mr. D. Becker for the statistical evaluation of the test results, to Mrs. C. Kirchner for her assistance in preparing the photographs and to Mrs. C. Wind for the expert typing of the manuscript.

Last but not least, I wish to thank the Deutsche Forschungsgemeinschaft, whose financial support made it possible to perform these experiments.

Homburg, May 1987 *B.-D. Katthagen*

Table of Contents

1 Introduction and Scope of the Study

Congenital or acquired bone defects are a central problem in reconstructive surgery of the musculoskeletal system. To accelerate the healing of bone defects, or to enable them to heal at all, it is often necessary to fill them with suitable, i. e. osteogenic and/or osteoinductive, substances. Because of their superior effectiveness, transplants of autogenic spongiosa, which can also be implanted if bone stability is lacking owing to the protective effect afforded by stable internal fixation, are usually preferred. Because of a series of disadvantages of autogenic bone transplants, which we will discuss in detail later, an intensive search for alternatives has been going on for several decades. In this context allogenic and xenogenic bone transplants will be mentioned first. However, for reasons of transplantation immunology and revascularisation, the effectiveness of allogenic bone transplants is limited, and that of xenogenic transplants is completely inadequate. Furthermore, allografts may bring hazards to the patient by the risk of infection (Hepatitis, AIDS, slow virus, bacterial contamination). The degree of care which is required today for choosing, checking and storing allogenic transplants makes this technique prohibitively expensive, and precludes its general use.

The "Kiel bone splinter" technique developed by Maatz and Bauermeister was therefore taken up with considerable interest. The transplant-immunological disadvantages associated with this material were thought to have been overcome by means of a special maceration process that did not affect its osteoinductive capacity. In the sixties, the Kiel bone splinter came into widespread use. However, in 1970 Schweiberer showed, that the Kiel bone splinter hinders rather than promotes bone regeneration.

Furthermore, Schweiberer (1970) made the following remarkable statements, which are summarized below because of their particular relevance to the matter in question:

1. Osteogenesis is primarily brought about by osteoblastic connective tissue that is not terminally differentiated.
2. Osteogenesis stimulated by the influence of degenerating bone matrix on mesenchymal cells has been shown to occur (osteoinduction).
3. Osteoinduction is not possible if the so-called unformed intercellular substances, the mucopolysaccharide complex, are removed from the bone matrix by maceration, boiling or burning.
4. The inorganic substances and the so-called formed intercellular substances (collagen fibrillae) present are of no practical significance in osteogenesis.
5. Bone regeneration is not accelerated by the availability of a basic structure, but proceeds along the vessels that develop from the recipient bed, and not along an artificial structure that is provided.
6. Macerated bone matrix is only slowly degraded by cellular and halisteretic processes; its ultimate fate is generally encapsulation as necrotic foreign material.

7. Furthermore, autogenic transplants are likely to remain the only really reliable transplant materials available that are able to initiate or strongly support bone regeneration or even to bridge bone defects.

In the 15 years which have elapsed since Schweiberer's publication, various authors have reported successful induction of bone regeneration using non-osseous implants. The implant materials used have been mainly heterologous collagen webs, decalcified, degreased and devitalized "bone matrix" and mineral substances, such as glass ceramics or various calcium phosphates. Reports of augmentation of bone regeneration by these substances are in complete contrast to the above-mentioned conclusions of Schweiberer. The bone-replacement materials mentioned above should therefore be examined very thoroughly.

In this project, we have compared different bone-replacement materials using the simplest possible test model which would, if possible, permit quantitative determination of the presence of regenerated bone in comparison to empty control cavities and to transplants of autogenic spongiosa. The aim was to determine whether these implants are of value as bone-replacement materials and, if this is the case, which of the materials are the most promising ones according to a quantitative comparison and are suitable for use in man. Basic questions about bone regeneration under the influence of inorganic and denatured organic substances have also been re-examined in this study.

2 Bone Biology

2.1 Bone Formation

Like all supportive tissue, bone tissue stems from embryonic connective tissue, mesenchyme, which develops from the middle blastodermic layer, the mesoderm, between the ectoderm and the entoderm (Blechschmidt 1960). Mesenchyme differentiates into connective tissue, fat, cartilage, muscle and bone.

A distinction should be made between ossification of the connective-tissue type and of the cartilaginous type. While the majority of bones are formed from cartilage, in the skull-cap bone and most of the facial bones ossification occurs with in the embryonic connective tissue. This process is called direct ossification. Osteoblasts line up next to each other, and secrete a layer of bone matrix. This process is repeated, and older osteoblast layers are at least partially transformed into osteocytes, and incorporated into the bone matrix, which then undergoes secondary calcification. During the process of bone growth, which is called apposition, resorption of bone substance by polykaryocytes, the osteoclasts, also takes place.

In the case of cartilaginous ossification, a hyaline cartilage of similar shape to the final bone is first formed and serves as a mould for the bone matrix. During further development the cartilage must first be degraded. The following sequence of events precedes this degradation: cartilage cells arrange themselves in longitudinal lines while simultaneously flattening to form a column of cartilage. The cells swell, and finally the cartilage layer is calcified. Degradation of the cartilage cells starts in the osteogenic cambium layer containing many cells and blood vessels, the perichondrium. This osteogenic layer contains numerous osteoblasts and blood cells, and is therefore capable of forming bone tissue. As a consequence of cartilage degradation, a cavity is formed, the primordial marrow cavity, which becomes filled with embryonic bone marrow. Endochondral ossification takes place primarily in this primordial marrow cavity, around residues of calcified cartilage. Cancellous bone is formed within the marrow cavity by interlinking of trabeculae.

At the same time, perichondral ossification proceeds from the residual osteogenic layer of the surrounding perichondrium. An outer cuff of bone tissue formed on the surface of the cartilage gives rise to the layer of compact cortical bone that surrounds the marrow cavity. The process starts at the centre of the diaphysis, and gradually proceeds towards the epiphysis, without however reaching it before completion of the growth phase.

Independently, endochondral ossification occurs in the epiphysis, leading to the formation of cancellous bone. Perichondral ossification plays a minor role here, which explains the thin cortex of the epiphysis. After the end of the growth phase, the growth plate softens, allowing direct bone contact between the metaphysis and the epiphysis, and thereby terminating longitudinal growth.

The perichondrium remains present as the periosteum covering the bone surface and as endosteum, the inner superficial covering of the bone. In proximity to the cancellous bone, the embryonic marrow remains in the form of red bone marrow. In the diaphysis, it is transformed into yellow (fat-containing) marrow.

The bones of an adult person consist mainly of lamellar, finely fibrous bone tissue; web-like, coarsely fibrous bone tissue is seen mainly during bone development. The osseous lamellae contain central vascular canals, so-called haversian canals, which are longitudinally oriented, and supply nutrients to the bone; they are surrounded by concentrically arranged osseous lamellae. The spaces between these lamellar systems are occupied by intermediate lamellae. On the interior and exterior surfaces of the compacta, the haversian canals are absent; the lamellae run parallel to the surface here, and are termed inner and outer basic lamellae (Figs. 2.1 and 2.2).

Apart from the haversian canals that traverse it longitudinally, the compacta is also crossed in a transverse or oblique direction by Volkmann's channels, which interrupt the lamellae in an irregular pattern and originate partly from the periosteum and partly from the bone marrow. Some of them terminate in haversian canals, and some anastomose with each other (Schumacher 1934).

Bone tissue is made up of bone cells (osteoblasts, osteocytes and osteoclasts), collagen and basic bone substance. The latter consists of organic components (proteoglycans, hyaluronic acid, glycogenic proteins) and an inorganic fraction, various calcium salts and water (Steinmann and Gitzelmann 1984). The mechanical properties of bone, hardness combined with elasticity, are due to the close bond between the organic and the inorganic components. The inorganic components are responsible for the hardness, the organic ones for elasticity.

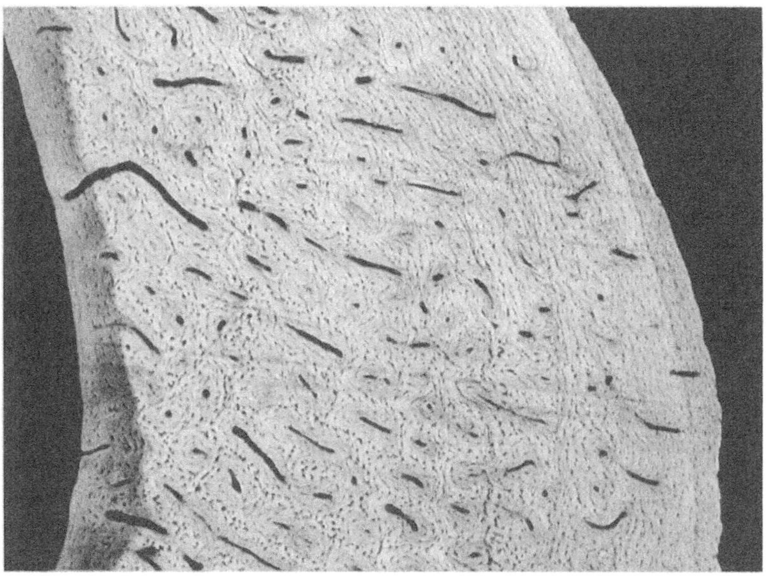

Fig. 2.1. Transverse microradiograph of rabbit tibia, showing lamellar structure of the cortex, with cross-sectioned osteons, haversian and Volkmann's canals. × 50

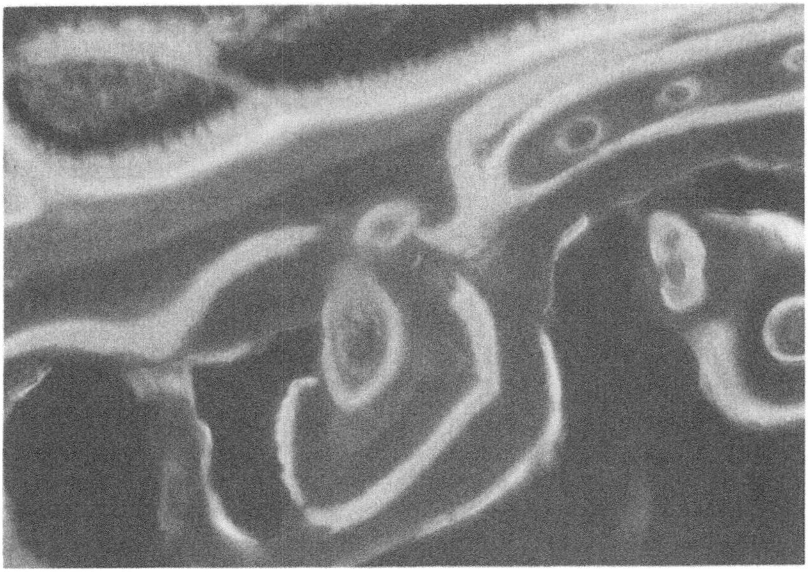

Fig. 2.2 Transverse section of rabbit tibia: polychromatic fluorescence sequence staining shows the development of osteons. The dyes were injected at intervals of 7 days. × 150

The elastic modulus of bone is of the order of 1.3 mN/cm^2, and is thus comparable to that of high-quality oak-wood. The tensile strength amounts to 17000 N/cm^2, and is therefore in the same order of magnitude as tough metals such as copper or duralumin. The compressive strength of bone, approx. 15000 N/cm^2, is much higher than that of many traditional building materials such as sandstone or shell lime. The static flexural strength even reaches values of 18000 N/cm^2 (Knese et al. 1959). These physical properties apply to lamellar bone.

The bone lamellae arranged concentrically around a haversion canal form a functional unit with it that is called an osteon. The average thickness of an osteon is approx. 3 mm; a length of even 7 mm is exceptional (Scharf 1960). The lamellar structure seems to be linked to nutritional requirements. The maximum diffusion distance is 200 μm for the spongiosa and 300 μm for the compacta (Voss 1954/1959, in Scharf 1960). Since diffusion can always occur from both sides of a bone lamella, the critical distance is 400–500 μm. Bone structures which are thicker than 500 μm therefore need intrinsic blood vessels that are no further apart than this. Haver's parallel-oriented vascular system probably represents the most efficient solution (Scharf 1960).

2.2 Bone Cells

The cellular elements of skeletal tissue can be subdivided into osteogenic tissue and haematopoietic bone marrow. It was originally assumed that these tissues develop from a common pluripotential mesenchymal cell. If such a common stem-cell exists at all, then it is present only during the early stage of embryonic development (Vaughan 1975). While the origin of osteogenic tissue is often attributed solely to the cellular elements on the bone surface and in the bone itself, recent investigations have shown that bone marrow contains cells which can differentiate not only into either osteoblasts (Friedenstein 1973) or osteoclasts (Hancox 1972), but also into haematopoietic cells as well as into any of the cells that originate from mesenchymal tissue. It is assumed that the haematopoietic stem-cells originate from the foetal liver, and are transported in the blood stream to the primitive, highly vascular mesenchymal tissue of the developing bone, where they form colonies; these haematopoietic stem-cells are thought to enter the foetal liver from blood islands in the yolk-sac (Moore and Metcalf 1970). The stem-cells then form actively haematopoietic bone marrow, which is partially replaced by fat cells, also of mesenchymal origin.

Friedenstein (1973) postulated the existence of two different colonies of osteogenic stem-cells, which he called determined (DOPC) and inducible (IOPC) osteogenic "precursor" cells. He justified such a differentiation with experiments showing that bone marrow implanted into a diffusion chamber was capable of bone formation without requiring the presence of inducing substances. The assumption that there must be a second group of inducible osteogenic stem-cells goes back to the experiments performed by Huggins (1930), who found that bladder epithelium which had been transplanted into connective tissue was capable of inducing bone formation.

In additional studies, Friedenstein et al. (1967) noted that cells from peritoneal fluid, which stem from the bone marrow, were capable of bone formation in the diffusion chamber under the influence of bladder mucosa. On the other hand, Friedenstein et al. (1968) found, in a similar experiment, that bone formation could not be induced with cells from different types of connective tissue. The differentiation of osteoblasts from precursor cells ("precursor osteoprogenitor cells") was investigated by various authors (Kember 1960; Young 1962, 1963; Owen 1963, 1970, 1980). Pre-osteoblasts could be differentiated from definitive osteoblasts. Scott (1967) also detected clear differences between osteoblasts and pre-osteoblasts using electron microscopy. The precursors of the osteogenic cells derive from a stromal stem cell, whereas the osteoclasts derive from the haemopoietic stem cell via a blood-borne mononuclear cell (Owen 1980).

By the injection of radio-labelled thymidine (thymidine accumulates in cells in which DNA synthesis is occuring), Owen (1963) showed that fibroblasts take up only relatively little thymidine, and play no part in bone-cell proliferation. However, a high level of thymidine accumulation was found in osteoprogenitor cells or pre-osteoblasts. These cells subsequently divide to become osteoblasts, which demonstrate approximately half the level of thymidine activity of pre-osteoblasts. Thymidine uptake also marks the incorporation of osteoblasts, and their transformation into osteocytes, in new bone (Fig. 2.3).

Osteocytes of different sizes and shapes, and with different intracellular components, occur. Jande and Belanger (1973) described three different phases: formative, resorptive and degenerative. In young fibrous bone, the osteocytes lie very close to each other, but are arranged irregularly; they are rich in cytoplasm, and can hardly be differentiated from osteoblasts. In the more mature lamellar bone, the osteocytes are flatter, and exhibit numerous delicate processes. The resorptive osteocytes are separated from their surroundings by a layer of amorphous material and loose collagen fibres (Vaughan 1975).

According to Matthews et al. (1973) as well as Holtrop and Weinger (1972), osteocytic cellular processes are associated with other osteocytes and osteoblasts. It has been

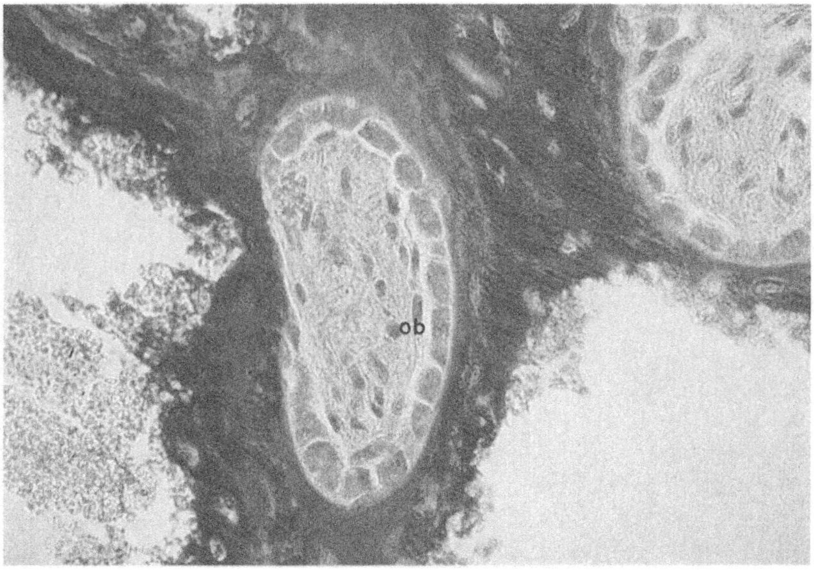

Fig. 2.3. Formation of new bone by large seams of osteoblasts (*ob*). The delicate osteoid seam and mineralized bone with occasional osteocytes can be seen; rabbit, Masson-Goldner stain (MG), × 250

known for some time that, along with the osteocyte, the bone also dies. Osteocytes are metabolically active and are involved in the nutrition of bone. However, osteolytic activities, such as bone-matrix modification and the dissolving of calcium salts under the influences of parathormone and calcitonin, are also ascribed to osteocytes (Belanger 1971).

According to Arnold et al. (1971), osteocytes work as "bone pumps", which drive water which has reached the perilacunar area along the canalicular network to the bone surface. This pumping effect is thought to be achieved via an osmotic gradient created by the transport of water-binding products out of the cells.

Bone undergoes constant remodelling. As part of this process, osteoclasts resorb residual bone (Fig. 2.4). Osteoclasts are large cells which can be found in the absorptive (Howship) lacunae, and usually contain about 10 to 20 nuclei. It was originally thought that osteoclasts were formed by cell fusion from special precursor cells or wandering cells, such as macrophages, histiocytes or so-called monocytes (Hancox 1972). However, the origin of osteoclasts is still uncertain. The osteoclast is a highly developed specialized cell, whose function is the synthesis and liberation of hydrolysing enzymes required for the resorption of normal calcified tissue (Doty and Schofield 1972). The mineral substances are possibly removed from the bone first, and the components of the matrix only then degraded (Reynolds 1968; Hancox 1972).

The enzymes cathepsin B_1 and collagenase probably share the principal role in the degradation of collagen, while citric acid and lactic acid are said to be responsible for extracting the apatite crystals (Vaughan 1975). Osteoclasts are influenced by parathormone, calcitonin, thyroid hormone and vitamins A and D.

The term "remodelling" refers to the process of resorption of old bone followed by the formation of new bone. Frost (1964) referred to two different types of remodelling:

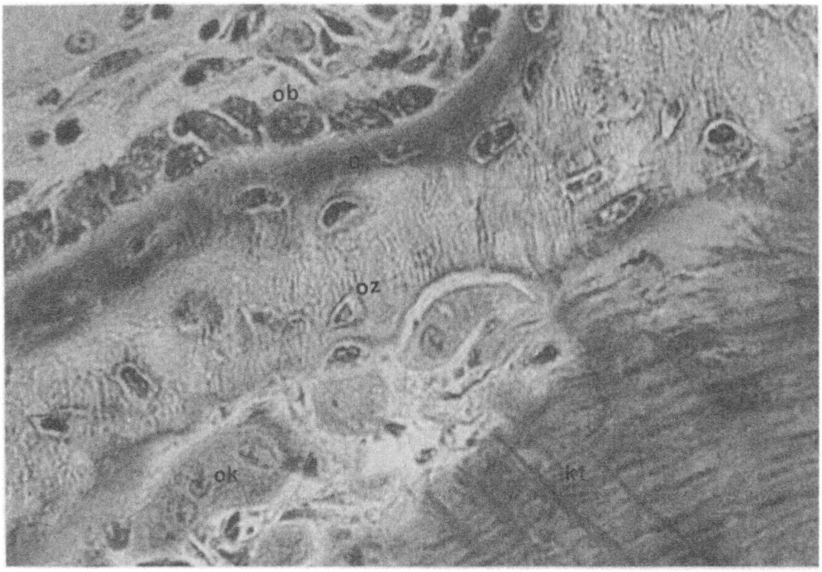

Fig. 2.4. Adjacent osteoclasts (*ok*) degrading a bone transplant (*kt*). Adjacent osteoblasts (*ob*), osteoid (*o*) and mineralized bone with osteocytes (*oz*) can be seen. (Rabbit, Giemsa × 250)

remodelling on the bone surface and remodelling within the bone itself. Bone degradation by osteoclasts is about ten times faster than bone regeneration through the action of osteoblasts; nevertheless, the skeletal balance between bone degradation and bone regeneration is about even. With increasing age, however, it becomes more difficult to compensate for bone loss, and the net result is a negative skeletal balance leading to osteoporosis (Parfitt 1984).

2.3 Intercellular Substance

The organic bone matrix consists of 90% to 95% collagen. Apart from the collagen, 1%–2% of the bone matrix consists of basic bone substance, which is made up mainly of glucosamine glycan and chondroitin sulphate. The remainder is made up of proteins, lipids and citrate (Petrides 1979).

Collagen is the most abundant protein in humans and animals, and accounts for about a third of the total protein mass (Neuberger 1955). It is characterised by very low solubility in the usual solvents, due to the presence of stable intermolecular cross-links. This makes it difficult to study its biochemical properties. The study of bone collagen has therefore been concentrated on collagen from chicken bone, because of its higher solubility. With certain restrictions, the results from these investigations can be applied to mammalian bone collagen (Miller 1973).

Collagen is made up of two α_1(I) polypeptide chains and one α_2 polypeptide chain, which are twisted around each other in the form of a triple helix. This tropocollagen is the structural subunit of collagen. Each chain has a molecular weight of approx. 100000 and contains about 1000 amino acids. The collagen molecule itself is approx. 300 nm long, and has a diameter of approx. 1500 nm. The three strands are cross-linked by hydrogen bonds (Shoshan and Gross 1974).

Glycine occurs at every third residue in the collagen polypeptide chain. Collagen also contains a high proportion of proline, hydroxyproline and hydroxylysine. The enzyme protocollagen hydroxylase hydroxylates proline residues that are located on the amino side of the glycine unit. The conversion of lysine to hydroxylysine is performed by another enzyme. Collagen also contains sugar units, which are linked to hydroxylysine. The peptide NH groups of one chain provide the hydrogen atoms for hydrogen bonding, while the peptide CO groups of the units in the other two chains act as hydrogen acceptors. The physical properties of collagen, such as its insolubility and high tensile strength, are essentially due to this cross-linking (Stryer 1979).

Larger precursor stages of the chains, the pro-α_1 and pro-α_2 molecules, are synthesized in fibroblasts and osteoblasts, respectively, and then secreted into the extracellular space. These precursors have a higher molecular weight, approx. 120000, as compared with 95000 for the α_1 chain. The additional peptide segments differ in amino-acid composition: they contain relatively little glycine, hydroxyproline or proline, and, in contrast to the α_1 and α_2 chains, they contain disulphide bonds. In the extracellular space, the N-terminal peptide segments are removed by a proteolytic enzyme, procollagen peptidase (Rich and Crick 1961; Kuehn and Zimmer 1961; Reich 1966; Hörmann 1967; Smith 1968; Stryer 1979).

Protein biosynthesis in cells occurs in the ribosomes, which partially line up against the endoplasmic reticulum and form polysomes with messenger RNA. However, occasional free polysomes are also encountered in the hyaloplasm. After secretion of the pro-α_1 and the pro-α_2 chains and removal of the N-terminal peptide groups – the role of these additional segments is to prevent premature fibre formation and to facilitate the transport of fibres through the cell membrane – the triple helix is formed in the extracellular space (Karlson 1972).

The above-mentioned smallest units of collagen, the tropocollagen molecules, aggregate in the extracellular space to form three different types of collagen. In the 280 nm-long "long-spacing" segments (SLS), the tropocollagen molecules lie parallel to each other with their ends level. In collagen fibrillae of the native type, with transverse striations at intervals of 70 nm, they are offset against each other by a quarter of their length. In fibrillae of the long-spacing type (FLS), with a period of 280 nm, they are antiparallel with approximately level ends. The lateral aggregation and the end-to-end bonds are thought to be caused by electrostatic forces which arise from the characteristic distribution of positive and negative charges on the surfaces of the tropocollagen molecules due to localised predominance of basic or acidic amino acids (Kühn and Zimmer 1961). Unlike bone collagen and connective-tissue collagens from skin, tendon and dentin, which consist of two α_1(I) chains and one α_2 chain, collagen from cartilage is made up of three identical α_1(II) chains (Miller 1973).

The tensile strength of collagen fibres is caused by cross-links between the molecules. Such cross-links can be formed between peptide chains of either the same molecule (intramolecular cross-linking) or different molecules (intermolecular cross-linking). There are few intramolecular cross-links in collagen. Generally, only one cross-link is found in a collagen molecule consisting of three peptide groups. When denatured, the trimer breaks down into a single and a double chain in a molecular ratio of 1:1. There are 9–12 intermolecular cross-links per mole of collagen (Hörmann 1967).

Cross-linking makes the fibres insoluble, increases their resistance to proteases, and considerably increases the tensile strength of the fibre protein. So-called telopeptides stick out like fringes from the rod-shaped molecule; they do not belong to the native three-chain structure, and are the sites of the intra- and intermolecular cross-links. Cross-linking of collagen molecules can be reversed by removing the telopeptides with pepsin or pronase. The native monomers of insoluble collagen can then be dissolved (Hörmann 1967). In bone, the collagen fibres form a stroma with a sponge-like structure.

The basic bone substance forms a gelatinous matrix which has an amorphous appearance when examined under the microscope. Apart from low-molecular-weight blood components, it contains mainly protein complexes with neutral or acidic mucopolysaccharides as well as glycoproteins and proteins. The insoluble precursors of collagen itself are also present in the matrix (Reich 1966).

2.4 Bone Mineralisation

The inorganic bone components, mainly calcium phosphates, which impart hardness, compressive and tensile strength to the bone, are incorporated in the fibrous collagen frame. These substances are necessary so that the skeleton can fulfil its supportive and protective role but at the same time they store metabolic calcium and phosphate under the control of the hormones calcitonin and parathormone. Calcium and phosphates are exchanged between bone and blood at an extremely high rate. Tests with radioactive isotopes have shown that 95% of administered radio-labelled calcium and 40% of administered radioactive phosphorus is found in bone 24 h after administration (Hayek 1967). About 29% of the inorganic phosphorus contained in rat epiphysis is renewed within 50 days (Dixon and Perkins 1956).

Crystallographic investigations of the bone minerals have shown that, apart from the main fraction exhibiting the basic structure of hydroxyapatite [$Ca_{10}(PO_4)_6(OH)_2$], bone contains further crystalline substances: octacalcium phosphate [$Ca_8H_2(PO_4)_6.3H_2O$], carbon apatite [$(NaCa)_{10}(PO_4CO_3)_6(OH)_2$] and brushite ($Ca\ PHO_4.2H_2O$). Apatite represents by far the largest fraction, and brushite and octacalcium phosphate are probably its precursors (Münzenberg 1970). These minerals are present in crystalline form. According to Münzenberg the crystal particles have an average size of approx. 9 nm.

Elliot (1973) published a comprehensive literature survey on the problems of determining the composition and structure of inorganic components in hard tissue. Reportedly, calcium phosphate can precipitate either in the form of plates 20–80 nm long and 2–5 nm thick, or in the form of needles. However, Elliot also pointed out the difficulties involved in structural analysis of bone minerals and commented that, although the structure of some crystalline substances analogous to those present in hard tissues had been determined, the modifications of biological crystals were still largely unknown. As an example, he cited carbonate ions. These were known to be capable of replacing phosphate ions in biological apatite structures but very little reliable information was available regarding their exact location and their influence on the rest of the crystal structure. It was also known that the different Ca: P ratios of biological apatites were due, at least in part, to loss of calcium ions and replacement of hydroxyl ions by water, but it was not then known which calcium ions were acutally lost and at which position the water molecules were localised. Also, uncertainties still persisted regarding the existence of different, i. e. crystalline or non-crystalline, phases of the bone minerals.

Young (1975) confirmed the existence of structural differences between natural and synthetic hydroxyapatite, comprising mainly CO_3-content, lattice parameters, water content, and the presence or absence of hydroxyl groups and hydroxyl-bound fluorine and chlorine ions. He concluded that it was only partly correct to refer to biological apatite as hydroxyapatite. The differences between biological and synthetic hydroxyapatite were more interesting and of greater biological significance than their similarities.

Regarding the contents of amorphous calcium phosphate, Brown and Chow (1976), in contrast to Harper and Posner (1966) and Tannenbaum et al. (1974), concluded that only small quantities of amorphous calcium phosphate were present in bone and, moreover, that the chemical and physical properties of biological amorphous calcium phosphate and synthetic amorphous calcium phosphate were different.

The ratio of the weight of the inorganic components in dried bovine bone to that of the organic components was reported as 77%:23% (i. e. about 3:1) by Carter and Spengler (1978). Collagen accounts for about 89% of the organic mass. Increased intermolecular cross-linking of collagen leads to a higher degree of mineralisation, and therefore to higher stability.

Microradiography of bone has revealed different degrees of mineralisation among the various haversian systems. Younger osteons have less mineral substance than older ones (Engström 1963). Apparently, the non-calcified basic bone substance, osteoid, contains substantial quantities of calcium in vivo.

It is not yet certain which are the important properties that a connective-tissue matrix must have in order to undergo ossification. Under pathological conditions, such as inflammation, paresis, trauma and the influence of tumours, ossification can occur in connective tissues that are not normally capable of mineralisation (e. g. myositis ossificans and periarticular ossification). It is not yet known what changes occur in the matrix or the fibrous structure. In bone, mineralisation of the osteoid formed by the osteoblasts takes place only after a certain latency period.

The transformation of bone tissue into a hard substance occurs only with the deposition of calcium salts. According to Eger (1963), the mineralisation of bone tissue is essentially determined by its neutral and acidic mucopolysaccharide content. Acidic mucopolysaccharides inhibit mineralisation by adsorption and blocking of calcium ions and by repelling phosphate ions. Neutral mucopolysaccharides, on the other hand, promote mineralisation by adsorption and accumulation of phosphates. Accumulation, not of calcium, but of phosphate is crucial for the mineralisation process. According to Eger (1963), calcium salts, including those present as hydroxyapatite, do not promote the formation and growth of bone tissue, but exert an inibitory effect.

States and Neumann performed investigations in 1958 with decalcified skin, dense connective tissue and bone preparations from calf, and were able to show that all three tissues were equally capable of inducing the formation of hydroxyapatite crystals from solutions with different calcium and phosphate contents. In contrast to the skin and the dense connective tissue preparations, however, only the bone was able to take up calcium from the solution.

Irving and Wuthier (1968) concluded that phospholipids play an important role in the processes of calcium-phosphate nucleation and mineralisation. If the lipids were extracted, the rate of recalcification of a decalcified matrix decreased considerably. On the other hand, if this matrix was then re-treated with phosphatidyl serine, the initial rate of recalcification was attained once more. Phospholipids favour the formation of calcium-phosphate complexes, and stabilise them. Inhibition of mineralisation by pyrophosphate was described by Fleisch and Neuman (1961). Removing this inibition with pyrophosphatases started the mineralisation process once again.

Termine (1972) described the process of bone mineralisation as follows:

> "At first, unstable amorphous calcium phosphate is formed, which is then transformed into carbon-containing apatite crystals, finally growing and developing into a more perfect crystalline structure. Interactions between matrix and mineral play a decisive role in this process, and the mineralisation has been described in the context of cellular processes."

A decisive step in the elucidation of the mineralisation process was the discovery of so-called matrix vesicles. These contain large amounts of phosphatases, and can therefore accumulate calcium and phosphate; inside or on the outer membranes of these vesicles, early mineral nuclei appear as needle-shaped structures under the electron microscope. According to our present knowledge, matrix vesicles are microcompartments, surrounded by a membrane rich in phospholipids (Krempien 1982).

Matrix vesicles were first observed in calcified cartilage by Anderson (1969) and Bonucci (1976). They were subsequently also observed in pathological calcification (Kim 1976) and in healing fractures (Lowe et al. 1983).

The cellular influence on mineralisation described by Termine in 1972 can be explained with these matrix vesicles, since they are highly specialised cell components. New osteoid can only calcify after a maturation process that lasts several days. The collagen becomes increasingly dense, the phospholipid content increases, and then 70% of the final mineral content is incorporated in a matter of hours. Further mineralisation follows during a second phase, lasting for months or years (Krempien 1982), which was described by Engström in 1963.

If glycosaminoglycans play any role at all during calcification, it is that of an inhibitor. While some investigations have been based on the premise that the apatite crystals are nucleated on the collagen, there are also differing views. However, it is clear beyond doubt that a strong bond is formed between the collagen and the inorganic components in calcifying bone (Irving 1973).

Boskey summarised the present state of knowledge about calcification in 1981. She described the cells in the ossifying tissue as the most important factor controlling the deposition of mineral crystals in the extracellular matrix. These cells are controlled by hormones and secondary messengers, as well as by other changes in their environment. They control the ion concentration in the extracellular matrix and the secretion of macromolecules whose properties determine the calcification capacity of the matrix. The cellular mitochondria accumulate calcium and phosphate, and release these ions into the matrix during calcification. Extracellular matrix vesicles play a role in many, but not all, calcifying tissues as carriers of the initial mineral deposit. Among the macromolecules which are secreted, collagen is the carrier for hydroxyapatite. Proteoglycans control the sequence and extent of mineralisation. Proteoglycans, glycoproteins, enzymes and collagen itself determine the properties of the matrix, while phosphoproteins and proteolipids may act as nucleating agents for hydroxyapatite. Finally, the interactions between these different factors control the calcification process, and determine the properties of the calcified matrix.

2.5 Bone Regeneration

Separate chapters have been dedicated to bone regeneration under the influence of bone transplants and bone-replacement materials. Here, we will discuss bone regeneration without bone transplants or bone-replacement materials using the process of bone fracture healing as an example.

Before the introduction of osteosynthesis into the treatment of fractures, only one type of fracture healing was known, the formation of callous. Willenegger et al. (1971) studied primary and secondary fracture healing. The following statements are derived from their publication:

Callous originally meant horny tissue. This term describes the entirety of all tissuerelated, biochemical and biomechanical processes from fracture healing to the final bony fixation of the fragments. The bulk of callous formation occurs in parosteal tissue, while endosteal callous formation plays a minor role. In the zone of contact between bone and periosteum new blood vessels and osteoblasts are formed during the first few days. In the vicinity of the fracture gap, the haematoma is replaced by granulation tissue and intermediate supporting tissue is formed. In the course of further development this granuloma tissue differentiates into fibrous connective tissue and fibrous cartilage. Both types of tissue are gradually replaced by fibrous bone until the final bony link between the fragments has been formed. The fibrous connective tissue in the area where bone regeneration is taking place exhibits a relatively dense network of delicate, voluminous capillaries, whereas these are virtually absent in the vicinity of the fibrous cartilage. This fact plays a decisive role in the ensuing ossification processes, since the formation of new bone requires the presence of capillaries. In ossification zones which are located in fibrous connective tissue, osteoblasts appear in the collagen phase, and are closely related to the blood vessels. They form osteoid, which then calcifies, and connective-tissue fibres are built into the new bone. On the other hand, bony replacement of fibrous cartilage is initiated by the formation of canals for the vessels. Importantly, ossification always requires the presence of blood capillaries.

On the other hand, physical parameters also play an important role; the zones of contact between unstable cortical ends are partially resorbed, and in the undisturbed areas distant from the fracture, lamellar bone predominates. The last phase of bone healing is characterised by remodelling of the fibrous bone and degradation of the callous.

With the introduction of stable osteosynthesis, a hitherto-unknown type of fracture healing became known, and was called primary fracture healing. This designation goes back to Lane (1914, quoted from Willenegger et al. 1971) and was later confirmed by Danis (1949, quoted from Willenegger et al. 1971) and by Bagby and Hanes (1958, quoted from Willenegger et al. 1971).

Assuming stable osteosynthesis, Willenegger et al. (1971) introduced a histomorphological distinction within primary fracture healing, between "contact" and "gap" healing. In contact healing, there is no space available for the penetration of blood vessels and tissue elements, because of the direct contact between the cortical surfaces. Because of this stabilisation, no shape-modifying resorption effects take place, and new, longitudinally oriented osteons bridging the fracture cleft are formed by simultaneous bone synthesis by osteoblasts and bone degradation by osteoclasts, which "drill" a so-called resorption canal. This leads to the formation of a bony bridge across the fracture cleft.

Gap healing takes place when the surfaces of the cortical fragments do not touch each other. In the presence of stable fixation, the gap is filled primarily by new bone tissue, and not by secondary ossification of intermediary supportive tissue. In this case it is essential that the bone cells are preceded by the proliferation of capillaries and the cells that accompany them. Krompecher (1937) mentioned primary angiogenic bone formation in the embryonic skull cap of the rat. Primary fracture healing corresponds to this embryonic osteogenesis. In gap healing, the fracture cleft is bridged by longitudinally oriented osteons only during a secondary step involving remodelling.

The prevailing biophysical conditions determine whether primary or secondary fracture healing takes place. Instability leads to the resorption of fragments, and to the formation of callous and fibrous cartilage; stability leads to primary bone bridging. In practice both types of fracture healing may occur at the same time, depending on the stability.

It is obvious that the defect size (width of the fracture gap after osteosynthesis) plays an important role in bone regeneration. Schenk and Willenegger reported modifications and limits of gap healing as a function of defect size in a paper on the histology of primary bone healing in 1977. They drilled defect cavities in rabbit bone cortex and observed the healing process. They found that bone regeneration starts immediately after placing the defect, i.e. without prior osteoclastic resorption. This finding needs to be specially emphasized, because it is often assumed that any bone regeneration is preceded by bone resorption (Frost 1966; Rasmussen and Bordier 1974). This statement was disproved by Schenk and Willenegger (1977). In the concluding discussion of our own animal test results, we will take up this problem again, because many authors have considered that inductive bone regeneration is only possible after bone resorption (W. Axhausen 1952; Schweiberer 1970).

Schenk and Willenegger (1977) found that up to a defect size limit of 200 μm, concentric filling with lamellar bone is possible, but that larger defects are initially filled by a trabecular framework of fibrous bone that is formed within 1–2 weeks. The formation of lamellar bone requires a pre-existing underlying layer of bone, which should be as flat as possible. For this reason, larger defects are first filled by fibrous bone, which is characterised by the absence of a lamellar structure; the collagen fibrillae form a random web. Fibrous bone contains many osteocytes, and is formed very rapidly; the interval between osteoid production and mineralisation is very short. This results in a broadly diffuse appearance with fluorochrome staining, which makes it impossible to calculate the rate of fibrous bone apposition.

According to Schenk and Willenegger (1977), fibrous bone is formed wherever rapid and voluminous bone formation is required, i.e. during the foetal period, in rapid periosteal thickening and during callous formation. They reported that during the first week defect cavities of diameter up to 0.7 mm were filled by fibrous bone, and that thereafter the intertrabecular space was filled by lamellar bone.

In our own experiments, which will be discussed later, it was particularly noteworthy that primary bony bridging of cortical defects in the rabbit tibia was only possible for defects of diameter up to 0.5–0.8 mm. After 3 weeks, larger defects showed a central area in which bone formation progressed only very slowly, and where intermediary connective tissue was also formed.

In 1978, Schenk presented a further comprehensive review of the histology of primary fracture healing. He underlined the differences between bone regeneration by primary ossification and the physiological remodelling processes occurring in lamellar bone.

3 Bone Transplants

3.1 Preliminary Remarks

The term "autogenic tissue" refers to materials which are taken from one part of an individual and transplanted to another part of the same individual. Autogenic tissue is considered to be the most suitable transplant material, because differences in histocompatibility and the risk of transferring a disease from one individual to another are nonexistent.

Isogenic transplants are materials which are transplanted from one individual to a genetically identical one, i. e. from one monozygotic twin to another. Allogenic materials are those which are transplanted from one member of a species to genetically different member of the same species. Xenogenic tissues are materials which are transplanted between individuals of different species.

The term "transplant" refers only to tissue, which may have been subjected to preservative treatment; it should not be confused with the term "implant", which refers to either denatured tissue (e.g. Kieler bone splinters) or synthetically produced or treated substances such as metal, plastics or mineral implants (Friedlaender 1983).

For decades, two conflicting viewpoints have dominated discussion of bone regeneration and the merits of different transplants. The osteoblast theory regarded a specific type of osteogenic tissue as initiating of bone regeneration (Ollier 1867; G. Axhausen 1908; Lexer 1911). According to this theory, osteogenetic cells themselves should preferably be transplanted, which is of course only possible with vital (living) tissue.

The induction theory is based on the concept of metaplastic conversion of undifferentiated stroma, but in the light of recent investigations by Friedenstein et al. (1968) it needs to be expanded to include inducible osteogenetic stem-cells in the bone marrow. The advocates of this theory claim that bone regeneration can also be induced with nonvital bone tissue.

W. Axhausen (1952) successfully combined both theories, in that he was able to demonstrate, on the basis of both the existing literature and his own experiments, that both approaches are possible. According to Axhausen, degradation of the basic bone substance plays a decisive role, since this process liberates substances which stimulate osteoblasts or induce the transformation of undifferentiated cells into osteoblasts.

Lexer (1911) pointed out another essential aspect of bone transplants, recognising the importance of the recipient bed. He classified recipient bed as being without, of weak and of strong regenerative capacity. Friedebold et al. (1963) performed studies which confirmed the important role of the recipient bed. Schweiberer (1970) described this in even more detail, and stated that under any circumstances the development of new bone in implant cavities always closely follows the blood vessels.

Bone regeneration under the influence of transplants or implants should always be interpreted as a series of events under multifactorial control. The implant and the implant bed mutually influence one another.

Disturbance of bone regeneration may be caused either by the implant or by the bed. Examples of disturbance caused by the implant are impaired vascularisation of the defect, immuno-defensive reactions and non-specific foreign-body reactions. Possible problems caused by the bed include inadequate blood circulation in the traumatised bone with devascularised fragments or infection of the bone. A spongy transplant bed obviously offers more favourable conditions for bone regeneration, due to the proximity of the red bone marrow with its abundant osteogenetic stem-cells, than does a deperiosteised, poorly-vascularised section of diaphysis. These factors will certainly have to be considered in the final discussion of our own experimental results.

The history of bone-transplant research dates back far into the last century. We will refrain from presenting another historical survey, and refer to earlier publications on the subject by Lentz (1955), Holmstrand (1957), Bauermeister (1958) and Schramm (1970).

3.2 Autogenic (Autogenous) Spongiosa Transplants

The excellent properties of autogenic spongiosa transplants have been known since the demonstration by Matti (1932) that autogenic spongiosa can survive transplantation. During transplantation, the more mature structures of the cortex and spongiosa become necrotic (Abbot et al. 1947). Maatz et al. (1954), who helped develop the Kiel bone splinter, showed, in experiments with dog bone spongiosa, that autogenic bone transplants are justifiably dominant compared to other commonly used transplant materials. Investigations performed with so-called millipore chambers (Segmüller 1967; Rüedi and Basset 1967) were important for assessing the relative merits of autogenic spongiosa. These millipore diffusion chambers were first introduced by Algire et al. (1954) and further developed by Rosin et al. (1963) for the investigation of bone development. The millipore chamber is a permeable container for cells, with a pore size of 0.45 μm. Tissues in the chamber depend entirely on diffusion for their nutrition.

Segmüller (1967) showed that autogenic tissue not only survives in these chambers, but also that fibrocytic tissue growing out of the spongy explants differentiates into all three supportive tissues, fibrous bone representing the final stage of development. Bony differentiation was seen in all experiments within 55 days.

Animal experiments performed by Graf (1959) with spongy bolts in spongy beds of adult dogs contradicted the above findings. Graf concluded that permanent survival of autogenic transplants was only possible if the blood vessels of the implant were able to connect to the recipient bed and that new bone formation and tissue development could only take place in an environment with functioning capillaries. This contradiction can be resolved if one considers that autogenic spongiosa itself is capable of bone production provided that adequate nutrition through diffusion is possible, but that with good vascularisation larger amounts of bone are formed more rapidly.

The significance of vascularisation for bone regeneration, which has already been discussed in the section on the role of the recipient bed, has been confirmed in more recent studies by Forgon and Bornemisza (1970), Schweiberer (1970, 1976), Saur et al. (1978), Decker et al. (1979), Albrektsson (1980), and Albrektsson and Lindner (1981). Albrektsson and Lindner (1981) were able to demonstrate by microscopy of vital tissues that transplants which had developed blood vessels at an early stage (5–9 days after transplantation) still contained living bone tissue and showed good vascular circulation

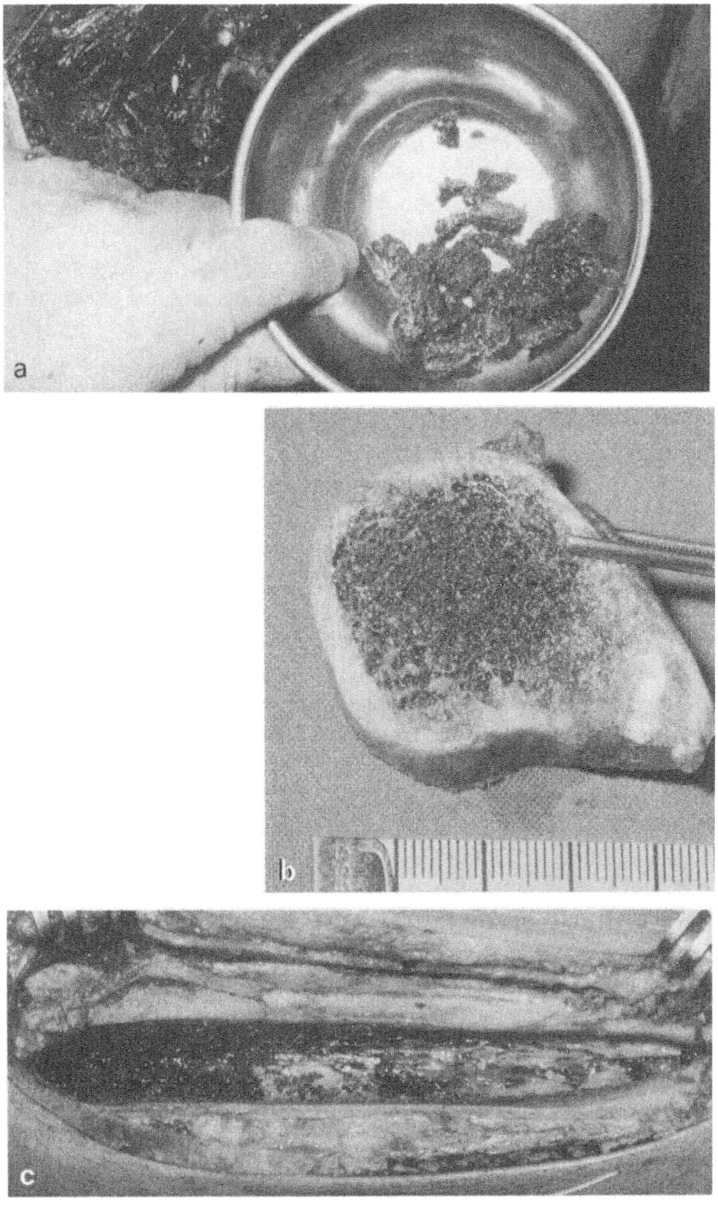

Fig. 3.1a–c. Autogenic bone transplant. **a** Spongiosa chips. **b** Cortico-cancellous bone. **c** Bone defect after removal of a large autograft from the tibia

after 1 year, whereas transplants which had developed blood vessels only after 17–29 days were only partially revascularised, even after 1 year, and still did not contain living bone tissue.

In summary, it can be concluded from the above experimental work that osteogenic stem cells can survive in an autogenic spongy transplant, and that the transplant itself has regenerative osteogenetic capacity. Because of the loose structure of spongy material, there is rapid vascularisation through the stroma, and autogenic spongiosa therefore plays a dominant role in bone-transplant surgery.

However, the real reason for the popularity of autogenic spongiosa is its clinical success in the treatment of delayed fracture healing, pseudoarthroses, bone defects and recently even infections (Schramm 1970; Burri et al. 1971; Schweiberer 1976; Decker and Müller 1980; Burri 1979; Müller 1981).

In view of the tremendous success of autogenic spongiosa in clinical practice, supported by the experimental results, it is not surprising that many surgeons use autogenic spongiosa and autogenic cortico-cancellous bone as their only bone transplant materials (Fig. 3.1a–c). Since – at least for adults – sufficient autogenic bone material is normally available for transplants, which is not the case for other tissues, one might think that the search for alternative transplant materials or for "bone-replacement materials" is superfluous. However, this is not so, for the following reasons: reconstructive surgery sometimes requires large amounts of transplant material, which may not be available in sufficient quantity, particularly during childhood. Some examples are: extensive bone tumours; systemic diseases involving bone destruction, e.g. cystic osteofibromatosis (Jaffe-Lichtenstein disease) or enchondromatosis (Ollier's disease); inborn or acquired bone defects and spondylodesis after correction of scoliosis. Particularly during childhood, the risk of damaging the growth plate during bone explantation should always be taken into consideration as well.

Moreover, the following disadvantages and risks of autografts for all patient categories must be mentioned: longer operation and anaesthesia, higher blood loss, risk of infection and, depending upon the donor site, risks of damage to nerves and blood vessels, thrombosis and fracture. Last but not least, the post-operative pain for the patient caused by the explant operation and also the additional scar, should be considered. Finally, the question of an osteoplastic replacement for the defect created by explantation in the case of large autogenic bone transplants remains to be addressed. Although autogenic bone can be obtained from the patient, this does not mean that there are no costs involved. The preparation of the donor site and of the instruments, drainage, sutures and dressings, personnel costs and possible prolongation of the stay in hospital need to be considered. There can therefore be no doubt that readily available alternative to autogenic bone is at least desirable for some indications in reconstructive surgery. This is also evident from the innumerable experimental techniques that have been designed to fill a bone defect and to stimulate bone growth with other bone-transplant or implant materials.

3.3 Cortical Autografts

Autogenic spongiosa has the disadvantage of lacking stability, and can therefore often only be used under conditions with stable internal fixation. At the beginning of this century, this possibility did not yet exist and the transplant itself had to provide stability in bridging bone defects or pseudoarthroses. For this reason, Lexer (1911) favoured the use of strong cortical autografts, which he notched into the bone as bridge-forming splinters in a carpentry-like manner with circular wire and screw fixation. The cortical splinter can be regarded as a rudimentary plate for internal fixation, which has, however, the advantage that it can still be resorbed or integrated.

Due to its poor vascularity, which, as explained above, is of great importance to the vitality of the transplant, and also because of its low content of osteogenetic stem-cells, autogenic cortical bone is much less important for bone regeneration than autogenic spongiosa. Cortical substance must either be completely degraded or be incorporated as non-vital material into the regenerated bone. Burchardt et al. (1975) therefore attempted to increase the revascularisation and thus the efficacy of cortical bone by drilling numerous holes into it. They found that although the holes were rapidly filled with regenerated spongiosa, this procedure did not accelerate remodelling of the entire transplant. Thus, the only role for free cortical autografts in bone regeneration is the temporary increase in stability obtained with cortico-cancellous bone. In the case of very large bone defects, the current approach is to anastomose the vascular stump of a free autograft to the blood vessels of the bed by microsurgery (Taylor et al. 1975; Weiland et al. 1983; Chacha 1984). Of course, the disadvantages of autogenic spongiosa mentioned above apply equally well to transplants of cortical bone and to cortico-cancellous autografts.

3.4 Allogenic (Homologous) Bone Transplants

The essential difference between autografts on the one hand and allo- or xenografts on the other hand lies in the immuno-defensive reactions that arise against the latter. The cellular elements of the transplant carry the antigenic structures; the antigenic properties of the matrix (glycoproteins, collagen and mucopolysaccharides) are not yet known in detail, but the matrix is species-specific and immunogenic defence reactions are not to be expected by the allograft matrix. With regard to these immunological processes, it should be remembered that bone is an "unstable" tissue which undergoes constant remodelling by resorption and regeneration. Thus, a foreign bone transplant can be incorporated into the bed by being degraded first and then replaced with regenerated bone (creeping substitution). In contrast to this, other tissues (e. g. skin and internal organs) are basically static tissues, which retain their antigenicity until total rejection occurs.

In 1959, Chalmers had already shown, in a large series of experiments, that bone contains antigens which provoke an immune response in the recipient. Since a latency period of approx. 5 days exists between transplantation and the host immune response, allogenic cells also survived, proliferated and formed new bone initially. However, after this latency period, the regenerated bone and the surviving allogenic bone cells were killed. On the other hand, the antigenicity of freeze-dried allogenic bone transplants was found to be lower. Chalmers therefore concluded that living allogenic material offers no advantages over preserved material; on the contrary, with regard to antigenicity, preserved bone material behaved more favourably. The proliferation of osteogenic cells observed by Chambers in the vicinity of the transplant was attributed to "bone induction".

Enneking also showed, in 1962, that allogenic transplants behave like autogenic transplants during the first week. Some of the cells survive, others die. There is vascular anastomosis between the transplant and its bed. In contrast to autogenic transplants, dense cellular infiltrates are seen around the transplant after 8 or 9 days, and the vascular anastomoses are obliterated. Finally, cell death occurs, both in the transplant and the tissue arising from its proliferation. Enneking showed that approx. 30% of allogenic bone transplants in rats showed the same immunological behaviour as autogenic bone transplants. He also showed that the bone cells were the main carriers of antigenicity and that the acellular matrix provoked a comparatively weak immune response. Thus, the hypothesis suggested by Medawar (1944), who demonstrated an immunological reaction to allogenic skin transplants in rabbits, could also be confirmed in the case of bone.

Najarian (1962) differentiated between the immediate and the delayed immunological responses. The immediate response is characterised by the appearance of circulating antibodies whose effects can be transferred to sensitized animals by the injection of serum. This is not possible for the delayed response to an allogenic transplant, but it can be provoked by the transfer of sensitised lymphoid cells. With allogenic skin transplants in mice and guinea pigs, Najarian found that rejection of the allogenic transplant occurs more rapidly when sensitised lymphocytes are administered intraperitoneally.

Heiple et al. (1963) studied differently treated autogenic, allogenic and xenogenic bone transplants in dogs. The graft was taken from the femoral condyle, and implanted into a defect in the ulna created by resection. They confirmed the superiority of autogenic bone; the second-best results were obtained with freeze-dried allogenic bone transplants. Regarding the bone-regeneration performance of the other graft tissues, the following sequence was established: frozen allogenic bone; decalcified allogenic bone; frozen, irradiated allogenic bone; freeze-dried, irradiated allogenic bone. Fresh allogenic, deproteinated xenogenic and deproteinated allogenic transplants gave the poorest results.

Langer et al. (1975) studied the transplant immunology of allogenic bone in detail. They detected no difference in immunological behaviour between fresh and frozen bone. The host tissue reaction, as determined by cellular infiltration, did not reveal any difference between the two transplants. Langer et al. concluded from these findings that freeze-drying was not effective to prevent immuno-defensive reactions.

From immunology, it is known that defence against invasive foreign cells also functions through cellular immunity mediated by long-lived, thymus-dependent T-lymphocytes, which represent the bulk of the circulating small-lymphocyte population. In contrast to B-lymphocytes, T-lymphocytes do not produce antibodies. Cellular immunity is therefore not transferrable by administering serum from sensitised individuals. The immediate allergic response is humoral in nature, whereas the delayed type of allergic reaction is cellular in nature. Sensitization of immunocompetent T-lymphocytes provokes a mononuclear inflammatory reaction, with cytotoxic destruction of invading cells (bacteria, transplants, tumour cells) and activation of phagocytic macrophages, which ultimately leads to the destruction of the foreign cells.

Bonfiglio and Jeter (1972) observed a reduced cellular immune response to allogenic bone transplants in rabbits which had previously received implants of bone-marrow extracts. They explained this finding on the basis of a blockade of the antigens in allogenic bone transplants ("enhancement"). Langer et al. (1975) also postulated antigen-blocking factors in serum to explain the diminished immune response to allogenic bone transplants they occasionally encountered in their experiments. Using the leucocyte-migration test, they obtained quantitative differences in immune response after 2, 4 and 8 weeks.

The observation by Enneking (1962) that 30% of allogenic bone transplants have immunological behaviour like that of an autogenic transplant can possibly also be explained by enhancement.

Veihelmann and Thielemann (1976) investigated deterioration following different preservation procedures by determining the activity of alkaline phosphatase. This method is expected to provide information about changes in the protein structure due to the method of preservation, since the loss of protein conformation correlates with a decrease in the activity of alkaline phosphatase. After preservation by deep-freezing, they found a considerable decrease in alkaline phosphatase activity, to less than half the level of freshly excised bone. Still, preservation by deep-freezing gave considerably better results than storing in Cialite or embedding in Palacos. In this context it is remarkable that "deproteinated" Kiel bone splinters still show minimal activity, which proves that deproteination is incomplete.

With regard to allogenic bone transplants, Schweiberer et al. (1981) reported that all the transplanted and initially proliferating osteoblastic cells of allogenic origin were destroyed by antigen-antibody reactions because they contained T-antigens. After this antigen reaction subsides, osteogenesis starts again, since an osteoinductive effect from intact bone substance still exists. According to the authors, there could be no doubt that an allogenic transplant had such an osteoinductive effect. In week 1 and week 3 after the allogenic transplant there was vigorous bone regeneration, while in the interim, an immune reaction took place. Schweiberer et al. (1981) claimed that the bone matrix was free of antigens. This is however not true in xenografts, since it has long been known that it is not only the cellular elements that have antigenic properties, but also the collagenic substances present in the bone matrix (Watson et al. 1954; Needleman and Stefanovic 1969; Steffen et al . 1973; Menzel and Steffen 1974). It is also wrong to assume that the immunological reaction has ended by week 3. Rather, the diminished immune reaction during this period can be explained by transient and incomplete blocking (enhancement) of the cellular antigens.

Elves (1978) studied the cell-mediated immune response to fresh, frozen and freeze-dried allogenic bone transplants with and without red bone marrow in the leucocyte-migration test and the "second-set" skin-transplant test. He concluded that only freeze-drying reduces the immunogenicity of allogenic bone transplants, while frozen bone, bone with the red bone marrow removed, and fresh allogenic bone provoke a cell-mediated immune response. However, since freeze-dried allogenic bone transplants lose their osteogenetic potency, Elves proposed that allogenic bone material should only be transplanted in the fresh state, and that immunological problems should be handled by determining the histocompatibility antigens and inducing immunosuppression. An immuno-defensive reaction to freeze-dried allogenic bone transplants was also observed by Burchardt et al. (1978).

The importance of revascularisation to bone regeneration has already been mentioned in the discussion of autogenic bone transplants. In the study by Forgon and Bornemisza (1970) mentioned there, revascularisation of allogenic bone transplants was compared with that in autogenic bone transplants. The authors concluded that, in allografts (unlike autografts) the blood vessels of the host stroma did not link up with those of the graft and that the blood vessels of the graft were probably destroyed in an immunological process. The revascularisation of allogenic bone transplants in the Maatz spongiosa test (Maatz et al. 1954) took three to four times longer than for autogenic transplants.

Dambe et al. (1978) studied the revascularisation of allogenic bone transplants in the dog long-bone diaphysis, using microangiography. In the first week, they found complete revascularisation of the allogenic spongiosa, but after the onset of the immune reaction between weeks 2 and 3, total vascular and cellular destruction of the transplant occurred. After the immune reaction had been subdued, a second phase of bone regeneration started.

In spite of the obvious immuno-defensive reactions to allogenic bone transplantation, this technique is used in clinical practice. Ehalt (1968) reported the experience gained with 1531 cold-preserved allogenic bone transplants within 18 years. He found an infection rate of 1.3%; amputations did not become necessary. In 88.2% of his cases, the allografts were completely successful, in 7.3% there was partial resorption of the transplant and in 7.5% of the cases total loss occurred. Finally, Ehalt considered that, from his experience, allogenic bone banks were justified.

Spence et al. (1969) found that, out of 177 solitary bone cysts which were treated by curettage and filling with freeze-dried allogenic spongiosa transplants, 55% of the cases healed completely, while 45% had a recurrence, with 36% having to undergo a second operation. In spite of this high relapse rate, they considered the technique of filling the bone cysts with freeze-dried allogenic bone transplants to be suitable.

In a later publication, Spence et al. (1976) described work with freeze-dried ground allogenic bone transplants, and reported healing in 88% of all cases. For this reason, they considered this material to be even superior to autogenic bone transplants.

In 1976 and 1978, Knöfler reported the results of 2439 allogenic bone transplants, mainly in children and adolescents. Indications ranged from osteotomies over pseudarthroses to include almost the entire spectrum of possible indications for bone transplantation. The infection rate was found to be 7.4%. The allografts were removed under sterile conditions from accident or suicide victims at the institute of forensic medicine and stored in a deep-freezer. There was no further selection or testing of the bone material with regard to infection or systemic diseases. In spite of his high infection rate, Knöfler concluded that autogenic transplants were justified only in those cases where the prospects for a successful allogenic transplant were not favourable (Knöfler 1976, 1978).

In 1977, Ackermann and Taillard reported 70 transplants of deep-frozen allogenic spongiosa obtained from the femoral head during implantation of a total hip. They concluded that in practically every case there was perfect clinical and radiological incorporation of the transplant into the recipient's bone, and not a single case of transplant rejection or elimination was observed. The risk of infection was not increased by transplantation. All things considered, they recommended allogenic transplantation. Koskinen et al. (1979) recommended allogenic bone transplants for indications such as treatment of low-grade malignant bone tumours. Popkirov (1981) described osteoplastic replacement of donor bone defects, created by removal of large quantities of autografts, with allogenic spongiosa. He reviewed 387 cases, and recommended the adoption of this procedure as a new technique.

In a very informative paper, Tomford et al. (1983) discussed their allogenic bone bank. It is interesting to compare the present bone-bank technique in the United States with those mentioned in earlier publications. Knöfler wrote in 1978 that the only investment required to set up a bone bank was the purchase of a deep-freezing cabinet or a medium-sized deep-freezer, and that the operating costs were minimal. In contrast, Tomford et al. (1983) discussed their careful selection of transplant material. The following basic criteria were used to establish the suitability of a donor:

1. No history of infection
2. Afebrile condition during hospitalisation
3. Artificial respiration not longer than 72 h
4. Sterile blood and urine cultures
5. No use of intravenous drugs
6. No steroid therapy
7. No hepatitis
8. No malignant tumours

A test for contamination was required for all excised bone transplants. Of 91 bone transplants removed under sterile conditions, only 57 were really sterile, while 34 were found to be contaminated, and were therefore useless for bone transplants.

It is also very interesting to examine Tomford's calculation of the actual cost involved, which included all the costs associated with careful selection, checking and storage of allogenic bone transplants and also included expenditure for personnel, premises and laboratory tests. According to the authors, the cost of a single allogenic bone transplant amounts to approx. $ 2500. Even if the costs of, and the care involved in, allogenic bone transplants in the United States may seem exaggerated at first sight, nevertheless the careful and thorough procedure followed by the Massachusetts Hospital is to be preferred.

If one looks at the 7.4% infection rate in Knöfler's patients and considers the social costs involved in a single case of osteomyelitis, saving money when choosing and preparing bone transplants turns out to be a very expensive decision in the end, quite aside from potential liability problems which may arise when infections, such as hepatitis or acquired immune deficiency syndrome (AIDS), or other transplant-related diseases occur. Since the beginning of this decade allografting has become more popular in North America and Europe. The results of osteochondral allograft resurfacing, allografts in tumour surgery and revision hip arthroplasty are encouraging (Friedlaender et al. 1983; Locht et al. 1984; Gross et al. 1984). An updating on osteochondral auto- and allografting took place in May 1987 in Berne (Aebi and Regazzoni, to be published).

In summary, allogenic bone transplants represent an alternative to autogenic bone transplants for certain indications. However, they require considerable care, involve very high costs, cause problems by resorption, fractures, and disease transfer and regularly provoke an immuno-defensive reaction, which limits their efficacy, the range of indications for their use and the availability of allogenic transplant material.

3.5 Xenogenic (Heterologous) Bone Transplants

The discussion of this type of transplant will be limited to a few remarks. It is widely accepted today that untreated xenogenic bone is an unsuitable transplant material for man because of the strong immuno-defensive reactions it provokes. Ollier, even in 1867, had already recognised the inferior properties of xenogenic bone transplants. For this reason, the immunology of xenogenic bone transplants has been studied by far fewer authors than that of allogenic ones has.

In view of this lack of published literature, Elves and Salama (1974) undertook a comparative animal study on the development of cytotoxic antibodies. They implanted xenogenic bone, both in the untreated form and after various treatments. In the case of untreated xenogenic bone transplants, all animals clearly had cytotoxic antibodies in the serum from day 6 after the operation onwards.

Various treatments have been tried with the aim of removing the antigenic properties of xenogenic bone. A prominent position is taken by the Kiel bone splinter, which has found its way into widespread clinical use after extensive animal tests, and which therefore needs to be discussed in some detail.

3.6 Kiel Bone Splinter

The Kiel bone splinter was developed at the Surgical University Clinic of Kiel in the early fifties by Maatz, Lentz, Graf and Bauermeister, and was approved for general use at the beginning of the sixties (Maatz et al. 1952, 1954; Lentz 1955; Bauermeister 1958; Maatz 1959; Maatz and Bauermeister 1961; Graf 1959). Bauermeister, particularly, performed many studies of different maceration methods. His conclusion was that oxidative deproteination with H_2O_2 and enzymatic protein degradation with trypsin was superior to all other methods.

The steps involved in the preparation of Kiel bone splinters are as follows: bone is taken from a bovine calf or a young pig, cut into a standard size and subjected to cursory mechanical cleaning, dissolving of haemoglobin in distilled water with several water changes during 24 h, deproteination in 20% H_2O_2-solution at 37°C for 48–120 h, hydration for 10–12 h, drying for 12–24 h and finally degreasing and sterilisation in an ether vapour steriliser for 12–24 h at 34.6°C.

The results of his animal studies led Bauermeister to conclude that these splinters were superior to all other known splinters with regard to tissue compatibility and osteogenic potency in beds of strong regenerative capacity and in soft-tissue beds, with the exception of fresh autogenic implants. However, it must be pointed out that the above-mentioned deproteination of Kiel bone splinters is incomplete, and that the collagen structures are basically preserved. According to Zitter (1983, personal communication), the Kiel bone splinter still contains 36% collagen.

The method developed by Bauermeister was also used by Schautz (1962) with allogenic bone material, and the preparation technique was again described in detail. Based on their own studies, Dahmen and Koch (1962) concluded that calf bone macerated according to the method of Maatz and Bauermeister (1961) was a perfectly useable splinter material which exhibited a good tendency to heal in. However, they pointed out the need for as intimate a contact as possible between the splinters and the bony splinter bed, since the implant can only be vascularised from there. Spongiosa splinters were better incorporated than cortical splinters.

Schilling and Nockemann (1962) were unable to obtain bone induction in muscle tissue, and saw only connective-tissue infiltration and ensuing resorption when using macerated xenogenic bone splinters. However, they reported better results in beds of strong regenerative capacity.

The first clinical results were published by Maatz (1959). His report was based on 141 Kiel-bone-splinter implantations, mostly with excellent success. In 1961, Bauermeister described the use of Kiel bone splinters for filling defects due to cysts, tumours and inflammatory processes in 34 patients, and Maatz and Bauermeister concluded in 1961:

> "In clinical practice, the splinter produced the results which were expected from it based on the experimental results (with only one exception – it proved to be useless in without regenerative capacity). In all other situations, it proved to be equivalent or even superior to autografts."

In a sample of 316 patients, the rate of infection in aseptic cases was 3.2%; the failure rate was 10.5%. Thereafter, the Kiel bone splinter came into widespread clinical use until Schweiberer claimed in 1970 (as already discussed previously) that it served no useful function, and should rather be viewed as an obstacle to the formation of new bone.

More recently, publications dealing with Kiel bone splinters have again appeared in the international literature. Salama and Gazit (1978) performed immunological studies after implantation of Kiel bone splinters in man. They detected some, although not very much, antigenicity of the Kiel bone splinter. Boesch et al. (1980) studied the combination of a fibrin glue with the Kiel bone splinter, and found an increase in osteogenetic potency. While Salama (1974) at first used bare Kiel bone splinters in man, he later (1983) reported clinical success with Kiel bone splinters which had been impregnated with autogenic red bone marrow, describing 110 implants in 98 patients.

In summary, one can say that the usefulness of the Kiel bone splinter is at least very controversial, even though limited success has been reported recently, and that, world-wide, it is hardly used any longer.

The next chapter will deal with the actual subject of this project, namely with bone-replacement materials. However, it has first been necessary to summarise the state of the art with regard to the different bone-transplant materials, since bone-replacement materials have to be compared with the other materials available and can only be discussed in that context.

4 Bone-Replacement Materials

Nomenclature

We use the term bone-replacement material in a broad sense to cover all non-osseous materials which are, or should be, implanted for certain indications (acute fractures, delayed healing of fractures, pseudarthroses, tumours and bone defects of all kinds, arthrodeses and spondylodeses) with the aim of promoting bone regeneration. These materials should, if possible, be only a temporary replacement of the recipient's bone. With regard to precise terminology, it would really be more appropriate to speak of "bone-transplant-replacement materials".

In a narrower sense, bone-replacement materials are implants intended as a permanent replacement for destroyed or resected bone (e.g. for artificial joints or compound osteosynthesis). These are mainly plastics, ceramics and metal implants, which will be briefly discussed initially for the sake of completeness.

4.1 Plastic and Metal Implants

The development of orthopaedic surgery in the past 30 years has been strongly influenced by the introduction of new materials (metals, polyethylene, polymethylmethacrylate, ceramics and plastics reinforced with carbon fibres) for temporary or permanent implants. These implants can provide temporary stabilisation of fractures, pseudarthroses and other bone defects; they can also permanently replace destroyed sections of bone. The latter type of implant is mainly used for artificial joints, in cases where the joint has been destroyed by arthrotic, inflammatory or tumorous processes, but also with compound osteosynthesis for internal fixation by means of a plate and bone cement after enbloc resection of bone tumours. The bond between the implant and the bone is established either by direct fixation in the bone, through indirect fixation with screws and nails or with a cement-like adhesive such as polymethylmethacrylate. This type of implant serves as a permanent bone replacement. These implants involve a series of biocompatibility problems, which can only be touched on by mentioning the key words "corrosion", "wear", "fatigne fractures" and "demarcation of connective tissue" (Harms and Mäusle 1980).

Because of the new materials available and the cement-free fixation technique for artificial joints, biocompatibility problems in joint replacement are now so far under control, e.g. for hip joints, that artificial joints can now be implanted in younger patients as well (Mittelmeier 1984).

Biocompatibility is less important in compound osteosynthesis of malignant tumours in older patients, since problems will not express themselves during the patients limited life-expectancy. Nevertheless, the problems of compatibility are still so severe, without going into a detailed discussion here, that except for the indication mentioned above, restoration of bone defects should be attempted with endogenous bone, which can be either transplanted or stimulated by means of transplants or implants. In contrast to the role of the plastic or metal implants mentioned earlier, this is the main function of the bone-replacement materials discussed below.

4.2 Collagen

Apart from cells and water, collagen and hydroxyapatite are the main constituents of bone, hence the value of examining whether they are able to stimulate bone regeneration. A fact that has been well-known for some time, and obviously speaks in favour of collagen as a filling material for bone defects, is the very strong haemostatic effect of collagen fibrillae. The bone cavities which need to be filled often bleed profusely from diffuse sites, which cannot be controlled by the usual surgical haemostatic techniques such as ligature or electrocoagulation. It was therefore an obvious move to try to use xenogenic collagen webs to achieve haemostasis and promote regeneration at the same time.

Xenogenic denatured collagen webs have been used as haemostatic materials for some time. Experimental studies in animals showed that collagen webs (Pentapharm and Braun, Melsungen, FRG), had favourable haemostatic properties which were superior to those of all other known styptic materials (Chvapil and Holusa 1968; Köhnlein and Mergard 1972; Hait et al. 1973; Haussmann et al. 1974; Vistness et al. 1974).

Moreover, a number of clinical publications already existed describing favourable local styptic effects of collagen webs in coronary and vascular surgery (Spängler et al. 1976; Abbot and Austen 1974), oral surgery (Hunt and Benoit 1976; Joos et al. 1979), plastic surgery (Riege and Köhnlein 1978; Priesack and Bohmert 1982), urology (Stockamp 1982), gynaecology (Daume 1982), neurosurgery (Schönmayr and Schepelmann 1982) and abdominal surgery (Fincato 1982; Funovics et al. 1982).

The biochemical processes involved in the triggering of blood coagulation by collagen have been studied in detail (Hovig et al. 1968; Puett et al. 1973; Wuppermann and Hörmann 1974; Balleisen et al. 1975; Abbot and Austen 1975). The conclusion from these investigations is that thrombocytes adhere to collagen fibrillae and continue to aggregate until a platelet plug is formed. Moreover, collagen activates Hageman factor (Factor XII), which initiates plasma coagulation, in turn leading to the formation of a fibrin clot. These mechanisms are of great importance for haemostasis in vivo. For instance, if the endothelium is damaged, blood coagulation is activated by the release of collagen from the vascular wall. However, for this activation process to come into effect, collagen must be present in its native triple helix configuration (Wuppermann and Hörmann 1974). According to Balleisen et al. (1975), it is essential that collagen is present as fibrillae. Dissolved collagen is less effective.

Contradictory information has been published regarding the activation of thrombocytes by the above-mentioned collagen webs. While Joos and Ochs (1979) described massive activation of thrombocytes with a solution of Pentapharm collagen web, Stemberger et al. (1978) found no effect or only minimal activation of thrombocytes. We therefore decided to study this question further with experiments of our own (Katthagen and Hellstern 1984). These in vitro tests regarding the effect of dissolved and undissolved xenogenic collagen web on human thrombocytes showed that the collagen webs from Pentapharm and Braun, Melsungen, do not have a collagen-specific thrombocyte-inducing effect in either the dissolved or the undissolved state. We attributed the haemostatic properties of these collagen webs in clinical and animal tests to a non-specific physical effect and possibly to contact activation.

In a comprehensive monograph on methods, results and problems in collagen research, Reich (1966) described the numerous applications for which collagen can be used in medicine. Chvapil and Krajicek (1967) described the principal medical applications as follows: vascular prostheses, haemostasis, suture, covering of skin defects and replacement of other organs.

Bedacht described animal and clinical studies on the use of xenogenic collagen as an implant in bone cavities in his thesis in 1969. He used xenogenic native and denatured collagen implants. In contrast to native collagen implants, which provoked extensive antigen-antibody reactions, immunological tests did not reveal the presence of any antibodies after use of denatured xenogenic collagen implants. After implantation in the bone cavity, Bedacht (1969) observed proteolytic degradation of the implant, formation of granulation tissue and the gradual replacement of this granulation tissue with new bone tissue. Bedacht considered that the proliferating osteoblasts extracted important protein building-blocks from their local environment to construct the organic bone matrix. He described the advantages of this implant as being: ready availability; the possibility of filling and modelling even large bone cavities; its porosity, which permits faster formation of granulation tissue and regeneration of connective tissue and bone; its favourable tanning condition, leading to a decreased resorption rate; its compatibility with antibiotics and the absence of detectable antigenicity.

In the early seventies, Benfer and Struck (1972) demonstrated promotion of fracture healing in their experiments in rats and dogs. Cutright et al. (1973) found that complete resorption had occurred within 40 days of subcutaneous implantation of an Ethicon collagen sponge, and that the implant was used as matrix for the development of vascular connective tissue. However, the reaction was accompanied by the formation of giant cells.

Cobb et al. (1976) implanted purified bovine elastin from the ligamentum nuchae and decalcified rat femur collagen contained in a nylon net into the defect created by removing the incisors in the guinea pig. They found that neither elastin nor collagen provoked an immuno-defensive reaction; bone healing was accelerated with collagen implants, but not with elastin implants. Springorum et al. (1977) found that collagen implants accelerated bone healing, in tibial defects in rabbits. Springorum (1980) confirmed this finding in rats, dogs and monkeys.

Joos and Ochs (1980) implanted collagen in the mandible, and found faster mineralisation and an increased synthesis rate in the osteogenetic cells, and consequently faster healing of bone defects. Krekeler et al. (1980) filled jaw defects in the dog with gelatin sponges and with collagen webs, and observed faster healing of the bone defect with the collagen web, but no favourable influence on the healing process with the gelatin sponge. Fabinger et al. (1980) also used collagen web in human mandibular defects, and detected a favourable effect on bone regeneration. The collagen web must be of high purity, because impure materials have an adverse effect on bone regeneration, as was shown by Weber in his inaugural dissertation (1985). Borckmann et al. (1982) studied the influence of gelatin sponge implants on bone healing in the dog, and did find a favourable effect.

4.3 Bone Matrix (BMP)

Decalcified bone was first used to fill bone defects by Senn (1889) at the Milwaukee Hospital. He prepared the material from fresh bovine tibia in the following manner: the bone was cut into small slices, the marrow tissue was carefully removed, and the bone was treated in an acid solution until it was completely decalcified. Thereafter, it was possible to cut the bone into small pieces of about 1 mm; the acid was removed by washing, and the decalcified bone was disinfected in an alcohol solution. Senn used this material for studies in dogs and also for clinical observations. He used the decalcified bone to restore the skull cap and fill bone defects in animals and, in humans, mainly for the treatment of osteomyelitis. He found that the decalcified bone was degraded by granulation tissue and eventually replaced by new bone.

However, the method was disregarded, and was only taken up again in 1965 by Urist. He cut allogenic bone into slices of 1–2 cm, decalcified the slices with 0.6 *N* HCl solution, then washed them with 0.15 *M* NaCl solution, and finally lyophilised them. Implants were placed in the rectus abdominis, quadriceps femoris and erector spinae muscles in rabbits, rats, mice and guinea pigs and in bone defects of 321 patients. Urist observed that acellular, devitalised and decalcified bone matrix (which is also called bone morphogenetic protein, BMP) was replaced by connective tissue within 3 weeks. Histiocytes, macrophages, small and large lymphocytes, and fibroblasts were found in this connective tissue. In parallel with the resorption of the decalcified bone, osteoprogenitor cells developed within 4–6 weeks, and between 8 and 16 weeks the formation of new bone was evident in 90% of the experiments. In the vicinity of the bone, stem-cells, osteoprogenitor cells and small capillaries could always be seen, surrounded by osteoblasts.

Urist also used other acids for decalcification but obtained the best results with HCl. He developed this technique further and later published new results (Urist and Dowell 1968; Urist et al. 1975). Different sized pieces of bone matrix were implanted, and bone induction was regularly observed, independent of the size. Urist explained bone induction with a morphogenetic charateristic of bone matrix that he called "morphogenetic protein". Finally, he used allogenic bone transplants which had been treated with chloroform-methanol and autodigested in phosphate buffer with iodine acetate and sodium hydroxide solution in order to remove the alloantigens while preserving the morphogenetic effect of the bone matrix. In this respect, recent results by Urist et al. (1984), which showed that a combination of tricalcium phosphate with bone matrix resulted in a twelve-fold increase in bone formation compared with bone matrix alone, are noteworthy. They indicate a synergistic effect of tricalcium phosphate on BMP.

Other authors subsequently also worked with decalcified allogenic bone matrix. Narang and Wells (1973) implanted this material into the root cavity of the tooth and also observed stimulation of osteogenesis. Plasmans et al. (1978) used decalcified allogenic bone matrix for ectopic bone induction in rabbit back muscles, and observed inhibition of this ectopic osteogenesis under the influence of diphosphonate. After withdrawal of diphosphonate, bone formation started again.

Tuli and Singh (1978) filled bony and periosteal resection defects in the rabbit ulna diaphysis with decalcified allogenic bone matrix. In 81% of the animals, complete bridging-over of the bone defect occurred after 12 weeks; local foreign-body or immunodefensive reactions were not observed. Tuli and Singh described bone matrix as a highly osteoinductive material.

Glowacki et al. (1981) also reported favourable results, in cranio-maxillary plastic surgery on 34 patients with 28 congenital and 6 acquired defects. Rapid bone healing was observed, and the advantage of unlimited availability was emphasized.

Chalmers et al. (1975) investigated bone induction with bone matrix in different soft tissues, and observed bone induction in muscle and fascia, but not in spleen, liver or kidney. When autogenic fascia was implanted together with decalcified bone matrix, bone formation was also induced in these organs. Heparin and diphosphonate suppressed bone induction. Chalmers et al. postulated the following prerequisites for bone induction in soft tissues:

1. An inducing substance, such as bone matrix
2. The presence of osteogenetic stem-cells
3. Suitable conditions in the stroma for osteogenesis.

In Germany, Thielemann et al. (1978, 1979, 1982a, b) worked in this field. They first confirmed ectopic bone formation under the influence of bone matrix implanted in the rectus abdominis muscle in rats, and later also regenerated resection defects of 1 cm in the dog tibia with bone matrix. However, only the allogenic matrix implant was successful and xenogenic matrix implants produced only inflammation. Osteoinduction was ascribed to a matrix-specific factor.

In 1984, Harakas prepared a literature survey on demineralised bone matrix, and presented a comprehensive summary of the present state of knowledge about this bone-replacement material. Because of the number of positive reports in this field, we decided to include this substance in our test series comparing the potential for bone-regeneration induction of different bone-replacement materials. Unfortunately BMP is not yet available for clinical application.

4.4 Glass Ceramics

The previous two chapters have dealt with the influence of denatured organic substances on bone regeneration. We will now turn our attention to a very different class of substances: biomaterials of mineral origin. To complete the fore-going discussion, and introduce the discussion of natural and synthetic calcium phosphates, which are of prime interest in this context, we will first deal with a further class of compounds, glass ceramics.

For this purpose, it is necessary to recall what was said in Chapter 4.1 about the replacement of joints with plastic or metal implants. It was mentioned that after implantation in the bone, these materials are demarcated from the bone by a boundary layer of connective tissue, which reduces the adhesion between the implant and the bone, and which may, under the added influence of foreign-tissue granulation and abrasive particles from the artificial joint, lead to loosening of the prosthesis. In order to solve this problem, researchers have concentrated their interest on ceramic biomaterials since the beginning of the last decade. In a review article on ceramic implants, Hench (1975) divided these bioceramic materials into three categories based on their biochemical properties: almost insoluble, very readily soluble and resorbable, plus an intermediate category. Aluminium-oxide ceramic, an example of an almost-insoluble material, was introduced as a gliding socket in artificial joints by Boutin (1972), Griss et al. (1973) and

Mittelmeier (1974) because of its high wear resistance. Calcium-phosphate ceramics, which will be discussed in the next chapter, belong to the category of readily soluble and resorbable ceramic materials.

Glass ceramics, which have been extensively studied, mainly by Hench (1975, 1980), Hench et al. (1971), Blencke et al. (1975, 1980), Schachtschabel and Blencke (1976), and recently also Eulenberger et al. (1978) and Raveh et al. (1982), have to be classified in the intermediate category. Hydroxyapatite ceramics, which will also be discussed in the next chapter, rank between the soluble calcium-phosphate ceramics and the bioglasses.

Chemically, the bioglasses consist of Na_2O-CaO-SiO_2 and P_2O_5. This glass-ceramic material can be regarded as biocompatible and biologically active, since implants in a bony bed lead to direct contact between the glass ceramics and regenerated bone without an intermediate layer of connective tissue (Hench 1975; Blencke et al. 1980). According to Blencke, the bond between the bioglass and the bone is caused by physico-chemical forces. A calcium-phosphate film and a layer rich in silicon dioxide are formed on the surface of the bioglass, and are thought to be responsible for the bone-glass bond.

In this context, Ogino et al. (1980) found that, with bioglasses which contain less than 46 mol% silicon dioxide, the calcium-phosphate film and the silicon-dioxide-rich layer were formed at the same time. With bioglasses containing between 46 and 55 mol%, the silicon-dioxide-rich layer is formed first, and the calcium-phosphate film later. Finally, bioglasses with a silicon-dioxide content of more than 60 mol% are no longer capable of forming a calcium-phosphate film.

Because of their relatively high biochemical stability in comparison to the easily resorbed calcium phosphates, and because at the same time they are biologically active, bioglasses have been recommended as surface-coating materials for endoprostheses (Blencke 1975, 1980; Fuchs 1983), as additives in bone cement (Raveh et al. 1982) and also as permanent bone replacements.

Just as bioceramic materials based on aluminium oxide, silicon dioxide and calcium phosphate are classified into categories of different solubility according to their biochemical behaviour, they also behave differently towards bone. While aluminium-oxide ceramics can be classified as inert, and an intermediate layer of connective tissue is formed between aluminium-oxide ceramics and bone, glass ceramics should be regarded as biologically active, since there is direct contact with the bone. However, hydroxyapatite, which will be discussed later, has even greater bioactivity. For this reason, we decided not to include glass ceramics in our experimental studies.

4.5 Synthetic Calcium Phosphates

The most thoroughly studied calcium-phosphate biomaterials consist of either hydroxyapatite (HA), with the chemical formula $Ca_{10}(PO_4)_6(OH)_2$, or tricalcium phosphate (TCP), with the chemical formula $Ca_3(PO_4)_2$, which normally exhibits the crystal structure of whitlockite. Tricalcium phosphates are usually implanted as polycrystalline ceramics, which have been treated in a sintering process (heating at 1100°–1300 °C) so that the individual crystals adhere to each other.

The first animal studies with local implants of tricalcium phosphates were made by Albee and Morrison (1920). They found this compound when searching for an artificial inducer of bone regeneration in fracture healing. They reviewed published studies performed with similar aims using various materials, none of which had given the desired results. In their experiments on rabbits, Albee and Morrison resected a 0.5-cm-long bone fragment from the radius, including the periosteum, and injected into the gap 1 cm^3 5% tricalcium-phosphate suspension, between the day of the operation and the 5th post-operative day. The contralateral radius served as a control. The tricalcium-phosphate suspension was prepared in distilled water, and then sterilised. While the controls needed 42 days on average to bridge the gap with bone, the fractures treated with injections of tricalcium phosphate had already healed after an average of 31 days. In a further test series, they injected the tricalcium-phosphate suspension in the vicinity of the radial periosteum without fracturing the bone. In this case they detected no stimulation of bone regeneration. The explanation they offered was that tricalcium phosphate in the soft tissues did not come into contact with tissue capable of bone regeneration.

In 1934, Haldemann and Moore repeated the above experiments with injections of different calcium phosphates, and discussed the literature which had appeared in the meantime. Eden (1923, quoted by Haldemann and Moore 1934) could not obtain favourable results with either calcium phosphate or calcium carbonate, which he used to fill resected defects in the rabbit. In contrast, Cretin (1924, quoted by Haldemann and Moore 1934) found faster bone regeneration with injections of various minerals. Murray (1930, quoted by Haldemann and Moore 1934) observed faster bone healing after filling a 2.5 cm bone gap in the dog radius with sterile calcium-carbonate powder and calcium phosphate. Rollo (1931, quoted by Haldemann and Moore 1934) observed faster bone healing in the rabbit with calcium glycerine-phosphate.

Injections of mineral salts into human fractures were also performed at the time. Murray (1931, quoted by Haldemann and Moore 1934) used powdered tricalcium phosphate and calcium carbonate, which was mixed with blood, to fill a bone defect in an infected tibial fracture; Cotton (1924, quoted by Haldemann and Moore 1934) injected calcium and manganese salts into some fractures, and Eden (1923, quoted by Haldemann and Moore 1934) even obtained permanent bone reconstruction in patients suffering from delayed fracture healing with injections of sodium phosphate and glycerine phosphate.

Haldemann and Moore (1934) administered injections of calcium phosphate, dicalcium phosphate, tricalcium phosphate and calcium-glycerine phosphate into resected defects in the rabbit. The contralateral side served as a control in each case. They concluded that monocalcium phosphate, dicalcium phosphate and calcium-glycerine phosphate had not a favourable, but an adverse influence on fracture healing. On the other hand, the presence of tricalcium phosphate favoured the formation of a bone bridge over the defect in delayed fracture healing.

In the course of further development, scientific research concentrated its efforts on different bone-transplant materials, until calcium-phosphate implants again became the subject of scientific interest at the beginning of the seventies. Since then, these materials have aroused the interest of not only dentists and oral surgeons but also traumatologists and orthopaedic surgeons.

Bhaskar et al. (1971) described implants of resorbable tricalcium-phosphate ceramics into the proximal end of the rat tibia. They found that the ceramic material was well tolerated, that the bone was deposited directly onto the ceramic surface, and that the ceramic material was phagocytosed by mesenchymal cells. Cutright et al. (1972) came to the same conclusions.

Getter et al. (1972) studied three different calcium-phosphate powders (tricalcium-phosphate ceramics, calcium phosphate and hydrated tricalcium phosphate) in the rat. The defects containing hydrated tricalcium phosphate showed the poorest bone regeneration; those containing tricalcium phosphate and calcium phosphate gave better results.

Clarke et al. (1973) implanted tricalcium-phosphate ceramics in dogs, and found bony incorporation within 7–8 weeks and a weaker inflammatory response than after transplantation of autogenic bone.

Köster et al. (1976, 1977, 1979) worked with compact cylindrical implants of seven different calcium-phosphate ceramics. They found that implants with 75% porosity could not withstand physiological loads after being implanted into bone defects in dogs, but that implants with 45% porosity could withstand physiological stress 8–10 weeks after the operation following a phase of initial immobilisation. They concluded that ceramic materials with a ratio of CaO to P_2O_5 of between 2:1 and 4:1 could be considered biocompatible. Later, Köster et al. also reported favourable effects when replacing conventional bone transplants with calcium-phosphate granulate.

Kallenberger (1978) confirmed the cellular and tissue compatibility of calcium-phosphate ceramics in rabbit fibroblast cell cultures, but the fibroblasts phagocytosed the ceramic particles and the cells died following intracellular accumulation of ceramic particles. However, this cell death was interpreted as the effect of natural cellular senescence.

Ferraro and Foreman (1978) studied the extent to which tricalcium-phosphate ceramics were resorbed after implantation in the upper part of the ilium in the dog. After 18 months, the material had been almost totally resorbed and only 15 vol.% of the implant as still present.

Snyder and Levin (1979) reported encouraging results with regard to regeneration using implants of resorbable tricalcium-phosphate ceramics after loss of the periodontium in 50 patients.

Shima et al. (1979) carried out cervical spondylodeses in the dog followed by implants of tricalcium-phosphate ceramics and observed compression with ventral or dorsal dislocation of the implants in 70% of cases. They therefore considered the implant material unsuitable for this indication.

In his survey on calcium-phosphate ceramics, Jarcho (1981) concluded that these ceramic materials have exceptionally good compatibility, both in the porous and the compact state, and can form a chemical bond with the bone in an apparently physiological manner. In his opinion, the available experimental and clinical studies showed that these materials possessed the potential for future clinical use as bone-replacement materials.

Kaiser et al. (1980) used tricalcium-phosphate ceramics clinically to fill defects resulting from cystectomy and root-apex resection in 66 patients, and observed an unexpectedly high number of complications. Out of 48 patients who underwent a follow-up examination after 1 year, complications requiring correction, such as fistulae, rejection of the ceramics or enlarged bright areas in the X-ray picture, requiring correction, were found in 34 patients.

Since these negative clinical findings conflicted with earlier results from animal experiments and clinical work, Wagner et al. (1981) performed further animal experiments on bone defects in rabbits, and confirmed the positive results obtained by other authors with regard to tissue compatibility, firm integration into the bone and resorbability. The explanation offered for the unfavourable clinical results reported was that particles from the previous root filler and, above all, silver shavings formed during the root-apex resection induced a foreign-body reaction. Insufficient primary stability and insufficient bone contact may also have been responsible. They suggested that smaller granules would permit more intimate bone contact and lead to complete bone reconstruction.

Driessen et al. (1982) performed mechanical, X-ray-diffraction and spectrochemical investigations on whitlockite sintered from tricalcium-phosphate powder and on apatite sintered from Merck apatite powder. These materials showed the same compressive strength (600 ± 200 N/m^2) as dental enamel. Whitlockite was unstable at room temperature under conditions of high relative humidity.

Flatley et al. (1983) investigated the tissue response to implants of porous tricalcium-phosphate ceramics into the rabbit vertebral body and the growth of new bone into the ceramic implant. Reticular bone formation was observed after 6 weeks, and lamellar bone developed after 12 weeks; the bone had reached the centre of the ceramic block after 12 weeks.

Aoki et al. (1977, quoted by Osborn 1983) reported that a certain fraction of the inorganic bone component consisted of tricalcium phosphate, whose structure was described as whitlockite. On the other hand, the structure of the high-temperature phase of tricalcium phosphate was defined as $Ca_3(PO_4)_2$, and exhibited orthorhombic lattice symmetry. He also argued that although the ceramisation of $Ca_3(PO_4)_2$ powder yielded the desired compacted material, the proportion of the material in the undesirable alpha phase increased as a function of temperature and that negative side-effects could not be definitely eliminated by modifying the phase of the tricalcium phosphate.

To summarise, the results that have been obtained with tricalcium-phosphate ceramics in animal experiments and in preliminary clinical trials can be described as showing: exceptionally good tissue compatibility, direct bonding to regenerated bone without intermediate connective tissue, faster bone regeneration and resorbability, but doubtful mechanical stability in the face of physiological loads acting on the bone. The difference in activity between the whitlockite form and the alpha form of tricalcium phosphate is of doubtful significance.

A certain amount of confusion exists in the published literature regarding the nomenclature of tricalcium phosphate and hydroxyapatite (HA); these designations are sometimes erroneously used as synonyms, although the two substances can be clearly differentiated analytically. In some of the publications reviewed below, it is not absolutely clear whether hydroxyapatite was actually used or whether the material used was not in fact tricalcium phosphate.

The first study known to us where hydroxyapatite was actually used stems from Ray and Ward (1952). These authors reported that synthetic hydroxyapatite was first prepared by Barret et al. (1951, quoted by Ray and Ward 1952), and that for this reason it had only been available since then. Ray and Ward (1952) implanted synthetic hydroxyapatite crystals into defects of the long bone in dogs and into cavities drilled into the hip and the skull in dogs, cats and monkeys. They observed that these hydroxyapatite crystals were incorporated into the new bone, were slowly replaced with regenerated bone, and obviously functioned as a matrix for bone regeneration. Relatively small bone defects were filled more rapidly under the influence of hydroxyapatite crystals than was the case for untreated empty cavities, but not as rapidly as cavities filled with fresh autogenic spongiosa.

Levitt et al. (1969) prepared hydroxyapatite ceramic material by hot-pressing, i.e. by simultaneously applying high pressure and temperature. Monroe et al. (1971) showed that apatite ceramic materials can also be prepared by the classical sintering process, i.e. not by the simultaneous action of heat and pressure, but by applying pressure first and heating afterwards. They heated the materials, which had been pressure-moulded from hydroxyapatite, to 1300°C for 15 h and thereby obtained a mixture of apatite and 30% alpha-whitlockite. By adding colloidal cellulose, which as burnt out during the sintering process, they obtained a porous material.

Klawitter and Hulbert (1972) studied the porosity of ceramic implants in some detail but they used calcium-aluminate implants. The results they obtained can certainly be applied to porosity problems with calcium-phosphate ceramics. They found that a minimum pore size of 5–15 μm was required to allow penetration of fibrous connective tissue; 100 μm was required for regeneration of mineralised bone tissue to occur, and 200 μm for the development of proper osteons. They also emphasized that adequate pore size alone is of little value if the connecting passages between the individual pores are smaller. The values just mentioned therefore apply to the size of the connecting passages between the individual pores. The larger these connecting passages are, the better the conditions will be for the growth of new bone and the vessels which it requires for its nutrition, but the weaker the implant will be mechanically. The authors pointed out that bone survives permanently only when it is subjected to physiological mechanical loads, i.e. it is otherwise gradually resorbed again. The implant must therefore also be capable of transmitting the physiological load exerted on it to the regenerated bone formed inside it. With a pore size of 100–150 μm, the bone had penetrated to a depth of 200 μm after 11 weeks and 500 μm after 22 weeks; with a pore size of 150–200 μm, it had penetrated 600 μm after 11 weeks and 1500 μm after 22 weeks.

Rao and Boehm (1974) analysed the influence of sintering temperature and sintering time on the density of hydroxyapatite. They found that the sintering time was not as important as the sintering temperature. The maximum density was reached after 2 h. With treatment 900°C the density obtained was approximately half that obtained at 1200°C. The compressive strength was shown to be an exponential function of density.

Young (1975) studied the differences between biological apatite and synthetic hydroxyapatite, and also the differences which arise when both substances are subjected to identical thermal treatment. As already mentioned (see p. 11), they concluded that the differences between biological apatite and synthetic hydroxyapatite were more interesting, and probably of greater biological significance, than their similarities. Differences were observed with regard to CO_3 contents, weight loss, lattice parameters, fluoride and chloride content, water content and also with respect to the content of lower calcium phosphates.

Skinner et al. (1975) investigated the stability of synthetic hydroxyapatites during thermal treatment in a vacuum and under atmospheric pressure. They observed that, whereas thermal treatment at 1000°C leads to some dehydroxylation but does not produce any structural changes, thermal treatment under a water-vapour partial pressure of 10^{-7} torr not only leads to dehydroxylation, but also brings about structural changes and formation of tricalcium phosphate. They concluded that the partial pressure of water contained in the atmosphere is sufficient to form the apatite structure even during prolonged thermal treatment at 1000°C. The stability of hydroxyapatite also depends on the temperature and the water-vapour partial pressure prevailing in the oven.

Ryshkewitch (1953, quoted by Peelen et al. 1977) described a method for preparing porous structures by the addition of different amounts of 10% H_2O_2 solution to the powder-water slurry. Peelen et al. (1977) adopted this technique for the preparation of a porous apatite ceramic. They described in detail the interdependence of the preparation process, porosity and mechanical stability. Porous ceramic material contains two types of pores. Macropores are formed by the addition of H_2O_2 during drying of the slurry at 80 °C for 16 h. These pores also survive the subsequent sintering process. The figure given for the pore size was 150–250 μm, but no indication was given of the size of the connecting passages, which according to Klawitter and Hulbert (1972) is such an important parameter.

Micropores (0.5–1.5 μm) are usually formed in the sintering process, and depend on sintering temperature and time. The total porosity, which includes macropores and micropores, is a function of the H_2O_2 concentration and the sintering temperature. With increasing temperature, porosity decreases, and with increasing H_2O_2 concentration it increases.

X-ray diffraction studies show that up to a temperature of 1200 °C the crystallographic structure of hydroxyapatite does not change. At higher temperatures, an increasing proportion of β-whitlockite tricalcium phosphate is found.

The compressive strength of these ceramic materials varies, as a function of the porositiy, between 30 and 170 MN/m^2. Peelen et al. (1977) remarked that calcium-phosphate ceramics therefore attain the same level of compressive strength as bone (40–60 MN/m^2 for spongiosa; 160 MN/m^2 for cortical bone). The resistance to impact also varies considerably as a function of the H_2O_2 concentration and the sintering temperature; calcium-phosphate ceramics do not attain the impact resistance of cortical bone. Apatite ceramic materials are considered to be long-term implants due to their low resorption. Flexural strength, particularly resistance to alternating bending moments, is therefore of fundamental importance for the long-term performance of the implant. Peelen et al. (1977) tested an apatite ceramic material with a macroporosity of 20%, and determined a flexural strength of 35 (± 10) MN/m^2, which is far lower than the flexural strength of compact bone, reported by Evans (1973, quoted by Peelen et al. 1977) to be close to 100 MN/m^2.

Peelen et al. (1977) also performed animal experiments. They implanted ceramic cylinders with a diameter of 2.5 mm and a length of 3 mm into cavities drilled in the rabbit tibia. After 1 month they observed regenerated bone between the bony stroma and the implant. The implant was in direct contact with the regenerated bone and not separated by an intermediate layer of connective tissue, and was being resorbed by multinucleated macrophages. After 6 months, 60% of the implant had been replaced by regenerated bone. Regenerated bone was observed in the macrophages and the resorbed zones of the implant. Peelen et al. concluded that apatite ceramics were good bone-replacement materials. This statement will be discussed in detail later.

Jarcho et al. (1976) chose a different method, described in detail, for the preparation of apatite ceramics. They improved the mechanical properties of apatite ceramics by largely avoiding the formation of pores, and obtained a compressive strength of 917 MN/m^2 with the best materials. Polished samples had an average tensile strength of 196 MN/m^2. Unfortunately, a more important parameter, the flexural strength, was not determined in this study. They later called the substance durapatite. In a later study, Jarcho et al. (1977) also investigated the biological properties of this material by means of implants in six beagle dogs. They drilled holes of 4.5 mm diameter into the lateral femoral shaft at intervals of 6–8 mm and filled them with durapatite ceramic implants in compact and particle form. The animals were killed after 1 or 6 months. At this time, the implants had been overgrown endosteally and periosteally with regenerated bone. The good tissue compatibility reported by other authors was also confirmed with durapatite. However, durapatite in particle form showed more bone regeneration after 1 month than compact implants. The authors explained these differences on the basis of mechanical factors; however, a more likely possibility is that the larger surface of the particle implant plays the decisive role in this context. Although durapatite implants do not exhibit significant porosity, firm incorporation into the bone was found, as in the case of porous implants. Jarcho et al. postulated a chemical bond between the implant and the bone.

Rootare et al. (1977) performed wear studies with hydroxyapatite ceramics. They found the wear characteristics to be similar to those of human dental enamel.

Osborn, Newseley and Weiss (1978), Newseley and Osborn (1978), Osborn and Newseley (1979, 1980), Osborn (1983) studied the use of apatite ceramics in periodontal surgery. They found that, among the available biomaterials, hydroxyapatite offered optimum biocompatibility, and that the material was only slowly resorbed. They suggested that the hydroxyapatite component also played the central role in the formation of a bond between bone and implant in the bioglasses described by other authors. To obtain a porous material, they adopted the procedure described by Ryshkewitch (1953, quoted by Peelen et al. 1977) and adapted to hydroxyapatite ceramics by Peelen et al. (1977). X-ray diffraction analysis confirmed the almost-identical patterns for synthetic and natural hydroxyapatite already described by previous authors. A study by Kallenberger and Schneider (1975, quoted by Osborn and Weiss 1978) not only showed no inhibition of cell proliferation by hydroxyapatite ceramics in cell cultures of explanted human fibroblast strains, but even found attachment of fibroblasts to the ceramic surface.

According to Newseley and Osborn (1978), the biological activity of hydroxyapatite ceramics depends on ion-exchange reactions in the adjacent tissue. They performed solubility tests after various sintering processes, and found that the leaching resistance of the ceramic material depends on the cooling rate after completion of the sintering process. The faster the ceramic material is cooled, the lower its leaching resistance. Apart from the chemical reactions on the surface of apatite ceramics, Osborn and Newseley (1980) later also mentioned piezoelectric influences. They referred to Fukuda and Yasuda (1957, quoted from Osborn and Newseley 1980), who found that hydroxy-apatite-collagen bonds form a piezoelectric element which reacts to bone deformation with detectable electrical changes on the surface. According to Bassett (1966) and Eriksson and Jones (1977), the formation of new bone is always linked to negative electrical charges on the surface.

According to Jahn (1968), hydroxyapatite acts as an amphoteric ion exchanger. Selective accumulation of calcium and phosphate ions occurs as a consequence of the negative charges on the hydroxyapatite surface. This leads to the formation of more apatite and stimulates the formation of new bone. Apart from the interaction between implanted apatite ceramics and bone crystals, bonding between protein molecules and apatite ceramics is also involved. Osborn and Newseley (1979, 1980) concluded that hydroxyapatite was an ideal biomaterial for implant purposes.

Niwa et al. (1980) performed a comparative study with injections of hydroxyapatite, tricalcium phosphate, aluminium dioxide and bone cement into the femoral cavity in rabbits, and observed rapid bone regeneration in the hydroxyapatite group, less regeneration in the tricalcium phosphate group and no bone regeneration at all with injections of aluminium dioxide or bone cement. They also concluded that hydroxyapatite is an ideal material for bone implants because of its good histocompatibility, marked promotion of bone regeneration and easy and unlimited availability.

Denissen et al. (1980) implanted hydroxyapatite ceramics into soft and bony tissues in the rat. In the soft tissues, connective tissue developed on the surface of the ceramic implant. With implants in bone, they observed bone regeneration and the formation of a very strong bond between the bone and the implant. In stability tests, bone fractures occurred, but never in the boundary zone between the implant and the bone.

Scan electron microscope evaluation of the interface between implanted hydroxyapatite and regenerated bone confirmed the direct bond in our own experiments (Brill and Katthagen 1987).

In summary, it can be concluded from the above studies that hydroxyapatite ceramics are biomaterials – with excellent histocompatibility – which obviously promote bone regeneration. Negative tissue reactions were not reported by any of the authors quoted.

Differences in resorption properties exist between tricalcium-phosphate ceramics and hydroxyapatite ceramics. Whereas tricalcium phosphates are dissolved and resorbed relatively quickly, resorption is considerably slower with hydroxyapatite ceramics. On one hand, the relatively rapid resorption of tricalcium-phosphate ceramics can be considered to be an advantage, because it permits the replacement of the implant with regenerated bone. On the other hand it is a draw-back, because as shown by Kallenberger (1978), overloading the phagocytic cells with calcium-phosphate components leads to cell death.

Other essential aspects of the performance in bony beds are the porosity of the implant and its resultant mechanical properties. High porosity is necessary in order to obtain complete bone ingrowth. Above all, the connecting passages between the pores must have a size (interconnecting pore size) of at least 200 μm, because otherwise the bone is only able to penetrate the surface of the implant. On the other hand, we know that bone is resorbed again unless it is subjected to mechanical loads. The efficiency of mechanical load transmission from the bone through the implant to the regenerated bone within the implant remains doubtful. The implant has inadequate long-term flexural strength, in spite of the high compressive strength and tensile strength for low-porosity materials. Implants exposed to long-term mechanical loads are therefore bound to fail when the mechanical load increases.

Therefore, for many indications requiring implants of bone-replacement materials, the ideal approach is not long-term or permanent bone replacement, but the stimulation of regeneration, in order to fill the defect with the body's own bone. Higher mechanical stability of the implant is a less important advantage, since it is bound to fail in the long term anyway, due to insufficient resistance to alternating bending moments, and preference is therefore given to the regeneration of endogenous bone. Where a compromise is required between mechanical stability and the possibility for endogenous bone regeneration, the latter consideration must have priority. This principle cannot, however, be adequately realised with the variably porous, but nevertheless compact, implants described in this chapter.

4.6 Collapat[1]

In 1977, H. Mittelmeier developed the idea of a new biodegradable bone-replacement material based on the main components of bone: collagen and hydroxyapatite. From the beginning, it was expected that such synthetic or semi-synthetic biomaterials would – just like bone transplants – stimulate granulation tissue to form new bone, and thereby replace the implant with endogenous bone tissue. Because of the substances used, the material was called "Collapat".

The starting materials used for the collagen fraction were two commercially available, purified materials of heterologous origin which were already in clinical use as haemostatic collagen webs. One of these collagen webs was manufactured by Pentapharm, and the other by Braun. Since these materials had already been used for years as haemostyptic agents, it was expected that no major foreign-body reactions would occur – in contrast to native untreated collagen of animal origin, which provokes negative responses and is therefore useless, as has been shown repeatedly in experiments and in clinical experience.

The collagen web from Pentapharm is obtained from pig skin, degraded by digestion with trypsin, dissolved, purified and finally freeze-dried. It is supplied radiation-sterilised as a soft flexible "foam". When examined under the microscope, the lyophilised preparation has the appearance of a freeze-dried collagen solution with meshes, whose gaps can easily be filled with blood and easily infiltrated by granulation tissue, permitting rapid resorption of the collagen material. Information regarding the manufacturing method of the Braun collagen web, which has a rather more fibrous structure, was not made available to us.

Since some experimental and clinical experience indicative of a promoting effect on bone regeneration was already available for collagen web from Pentapharm (Springorum et al. 1977; Springorum 1980; Joos et al. 1979; Joos and Ochs 1980), and since this material seemed more suitable as a carrier for granular apatite because of its more net-like structure, we finally decided to use the Pentapharm collagen web for Collapat.

With respect to the mineral components, it appeared reasonable at first to use synthetic calcium phosphates such as hydroxyapatite, since some of these materials are commercially available at relatively low cost. In particular, we used a preparation from Merck sold under the designation "tricalcium phosphate" (pentacalcium-phosphate hydroxyl), which up to then had been produced for other purposes (the main technical use for hydroxyapatite was as a carrier in chromatographic analysis of chemicals).

Based on information obtained from the company and from our own animal experiments and X-ray crystallographic investigations, it became apparent that the material was until then not supplied in a constant composition, but with a Ca-P ratio which sometimes corresponded to a higher proportion of tricalcium phosphate and sometimes to more hydroxyapatite. As will be discussed later, a batch containing mostly hydroxyapatite and only a small amount of tricalcium phosphate is more favourable than a batch with a higher content of tricalcium phosphate. The hydroxyapatite content is of the order of 90%, which according to Petrides (1979) also applies to natural bone tissue. The commercially available mineral powder consists of crystals which are mostly smaller

[1] Manufacturer: Osteo AG

than 20 μm. It is off-white in colour, and tends to agglomerate. It was initially used in its native form, i.e. as a powder.

For histological evaluation of the basic components and particularly of the formulated preparations used in animal experiments, a modification of the cavity test developed in the dog by Maatz et al. (1954), and also used by Schweiberer (1970), was used. The cavities were placed in the rabbit femoral condyle, which has many advantages. The method will be described in detail in the Sect. 5. It was found to be very suitable for quantitative histological evaluation of the basic components and biomaterials used in animal experiments. The possibility of performing a control experiment by simultaneously placing a defect on the contralateral side proved to be a special advantage of the test system, particularly when the control cavity in the opposite limb was left open to show uninfluenced, natural bone regeneration.

Nizard's initial investigations (1981) first showed that uninfluenced healing of the defect cavity generally leads predominantly to marrow regeneration, and that only a little bone regeneration at the edges occurs. When collagen webs were used, there was also an initial strong macrophagocytic resorption phase followed by regeneration of the defect, predominantly with marrow; bone regeneration was observed only at the edges in most instances. The strong osteoregenerative effect reported by other authors could not be confirmed.

Problems caused by washing out and sedimentation were encountered with implants of apatite powder when the cavities are not filled uniformly, but at the edges of the powder conglomerations remarkable and unequivocal osteogeneration was observed, sometimes even with cross-linking. A somewhat better but still unsatisfactory and non-uniform apatite distribution was obtained with manually formulated mixed preparations (Collapat A). However, with this material as well, there was clear osteoregeneration around the apatite particles with partial cross-linking and new bone formation, whereas in the areas containing only collagen web there was no obvious formation of new bone, except at the edges.

These fundamental qualitative studies made it clear beyond question that apatite stimulates bone tissue far more potently than collagen does, and that what was therefore required was to ensure the homogeneous distribution of sufficiently large quantities of apatite within the collagen. Accordingly, the next stage was to attempt to stir the apatite powder into the collagen solution before lyophilisation, i.e. in the wet phase, in a ratio of 2:1 (Collapat B). Nizzard (1981) performed only a few experiments with this material, which looked promising with regard to bone regeneration, but was not yet satisfactory in our own experiments described below. As will be explained in detail, apatite in a weight ratio of 2:1 in the form of finely dispersed, small, powdery particles is obviously not sufficiently effective.

Mittelmeier therefore decided to increase the apatite concentration to a ratio of 5:1 with respect to the collagen carrier medium, and at the same time to concentrate the powdery apatite particles by transforming them into ceramised granules (Apagran). The ceramised granules were intended to act as a "massive charge" on osteoregeneration, as had initially been observed for the powder conglomerates in tests with dry mixtures (Collapat A). This stage was called Collapat D. (The modified product Collapat C was found to be inadequate from the beginning, and was therefore not pursued further.) Experiments with ceramised apatite granules (Apagran) and with Collapat D formed part of the present project, and produced excellent bone-regeneration results in animal tests, far superior to the results seen with earlier products with regard to quantity and homogeneity.

Collapat A, B, and D were also subjected to clinical tests for appropriate indications, partly revealing good osteoregeneration; in particular, no adverse effects, either general or local, were reported. The only somewhat-unfavourable aspect was that in larger implants the collagen fleece dissolved prematurely, due to its solubility, before structural stabilisation of the tissue could take place, which resulted in sedimentation of the apatite. To overcome this difficulty, the dissolved collagen was subjected, in a further stage, to a chemical re-cross-linking process in the wet phase by substoichiometric treatment with formaldehyde. In this way, dissolved molecular collagen is again transformed into larger collagen complexes, which no longer dissolve in aqueous fluids, but maintain their gelatinous consistency. With this technique, the capacity to carry ceramised apatite granules could be increased considerably until sufficient tissue stabilisation developed. The cross-linking with formaldehyde was performed in such a manner that CH_2 links were formed between the collagen molecules, with the liberation of 1 mole H_2O and total consumption of formaldehyde, which was present in substoichiometric amounts. Genius (personal communication) demonstrated that Collapat treated according to this procedure did not contain any residual formaldehyde.

The final stage of development, which was called Collapat E, consisted of finely dispersed, ceramised apatite granules with a significantly higher effectiveness, which are mixed with, and homogeneously distributed in, purified and re-cross-linked collagen web (as carrier material) in a ratio of 5:1. Our subsequent animal experiments, which we will discuss below, showed that this product is ideally suited for the realisation of Mittelmeier's concept of multicentric bone regeneration around dispersed hydroxyapatite particles [Katthagen and Mittelmeier 1984]. The easily resorbable, immunogen-free collagen substance permits rapid and unimpeded invasion by granulation tissue, and under the biochemical influence of hydroxyapatite a dense network of endogenous regenerated bone soon develops on the surface of the granulation tissue and in the gaps between the meshes, which were initially partly filled with collagen. In contrast to the entirely qualitative approach used in Nizard's investigations (1981), this project introduces a quantitative assessment of bone regeneration, primarily by means of accurate histomorphometric evaluation, thereby allowing quantitative comparison with natural, uninfluenced bone healing and other substances used for bone regeneration.

The final product developed in the Collapat series (Collapat E) is now manufactured industrially and available under the trade name Collapat. The product is presently undergoing extended clinical trials. Approval for general use, by the respective regulatory authorities, can be expected shortly.

Collapat was first mentioned in the literature in 1981 (Mittelmeier and Nizard). The animal experiments regarding the effects of collagen webs, hydroxyapatite and the dry-mixed preparations (Collapat A), as well as the initial pilot studies with Collapat B, were published in Nizard's thesis (1981). This publication also reported the first uses in man. Further publications by Mittelmeier and Nizard appeared in 1982 and 1983; in particular, Mittelmeier and Katthagen (1983) reported on the experience gained with the use of Collapat in 94 implants on 85 patients. In the meantime, experience has been gained from use in over 250 patients (Fig. 4.1).

With respect to indications for Collapat, it must be borne in mind that the preparation has so far been tested only in recipient beds of strong regenerative capacity, i.e. in

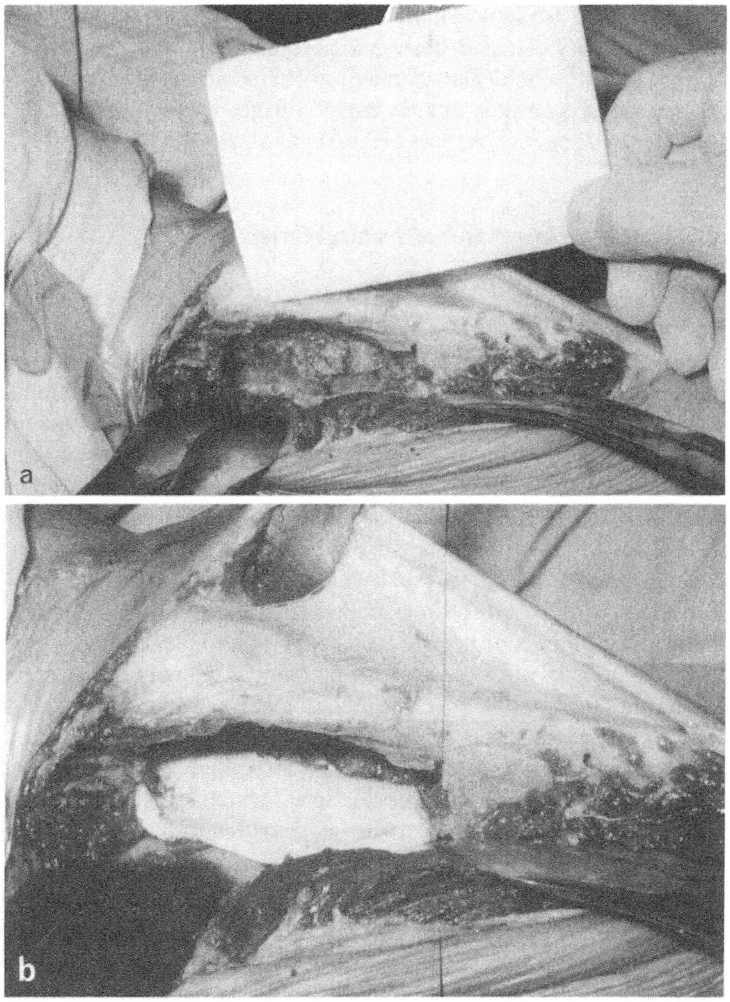

Fig. 4.1a, b. Clinical result after filling a bone defect with Collapat. The material can be modelled easily, has a styptic effect, and promotes bone regeneration

contact with bone tissue (in bone cavities and on the bone surface). Beds of low regenerative capacity have not yet been sufficiently investigated. Accordingly, the use of Collapat for bone regeneration is only recommended in beds of high regenerative capacity. The principal applications are the filling of bone defects after excision of autografts, the filling of benign cystic tumour defects, large spondylodeses in cases of scoliosis (Harrington), fractures and similar uses. Mixing with autogenic bone (augmentation) is also recommended. However, it has to be remembered that Collapat does not have pressure stability or dimensional stability. For reasons of safety, it must therefore be used in combination with stable bone residues, internal fixation or stabilising cortico-cancellous grafts. Because of this, we consider that for wide defects, such as defect pseudarthroses, elongation osteotomies, reconstruction after total bone resection of tumours, etc., Collapat alone is not sufficient and should only be used in combination with temporary osteosyntheses and autografts.

Finally, we would like to mention that polycentric bone regeneration with a fine dispersion of synthetic apatite using collagen as the carrier has also been attempted recently by Japanese authors (Hayashi et al. 1982).

4.7 Calcium Phosphates of Natural Origin

Besides the experiments aiming to stimulate bone regeneration with synthetic calcium phosphates described in the previous chapter, earlier experiments attempted to achieve the same effect with natural calcium phosphates. The materials used were natural bone mineral, and calcium phosphates or calcium carbonates obtained from corals.

To obtain a pure form of the natural bone mineral, it is necessary to remove all organic components completely, i. e. cells, fat, collagenous structures and unformed intercellular substance. As mentioned earlier, the Kiel bone splinter is only incompletely deproteinated, and the collagen in the matrix is largely preserved. According to Bauermeister (1958), attempts to remove all organic materials completely by boiling have either yielded good maceration results but at the same time destroyed most of the hard substance, or else given only moderate maceration while leaving the hard substance intact. The process of boiling attacks the mineral substance so strongly that no usable material remains after completely removing all the organic structures.

Further studies took the approach of burning the organic substances (Ollier 1858, quoted by Bauermeister 1958; Landerer 1895, quoted by Bauermeister 1958; Marchand 1899; Orell 1934; Maatz 1951, 1954, quoted by Bauermeister 1958; Holmstand 1957; Osborn 1983, personal communication). Marchand and Orell had already noted that when bone was burnt, the soft tissue was often only charred, and plugged up the tiny canals, creating a chemical and mechanical obstacle to the penetration of granuloma tissue. Maatz therefore tried prior maceration by boiling with bicarbonate solution. Bauermeister concluded that this method was really only of theoretical interest, since the mechanical stability of the bone splinter was almost totally destroyed by burning, and the material could therefore no longer be used as an implant where there was a need for mechanical stability. He commented that the mechanical stability of the splinters was totally destroyed, and that they crumbled when held in the open hand. Bauermeister (1958) even asserted that conventionally burnt splinters also lost their osteogenic momentum because of a change in crystal structure during the burning process. In his opinion, the "osteoinductive" potency of the splinters depended on the presence of an intact crystalline structure, which should therefore not be changed during the process. Osborn also expressed the opinion recently that maceration by burning produces splinter material that is unusable for mechanical reasons.

A study reported by Losel and Hurley (1958, quoted by Basset et al. 1962), who found no immune response and rapid new-bone penetration using inorganic bone, prompted Basset et al. (1962) to investigate the long-term behaviour of inorganic bone implants, which were however of cortical origin. They concluded that 80% of the implant was still present after 1 year, and that replacement by endogenous bone proceeded extremely slowly. This would inhibit natural bone remodelling. For this reason, and also because of its fragility, inorganic bone has rightly been considered unsuitable for use in man.

Schweiberer (1970) also worked with pre-macerated bone, which he incinerated in a quartz oven. He was able to provoke a marked connective-tissue reaction, but observed no acceleration of osteogenesis by the calcium-salt matrix.

How is it then possible to explain the discrepancy between the favourable results obtained with synthetically manufactured calcium-phosphate ceramic materials and the discouraging results seen with mineral materials obtained from natural bone by burning off the organic components, which also consist mainly of hydroxyapatite? In the burning process described by the above authors, some of the organic components are only charred, and hence remain in this form in the mineral structure, masking it, and provoking a severe immuno-defensive reaction against the foreign material. Moreover, when bone, which still contains water and organic material, is treated in a burning process, this necessarily results in an almost explosive vaporisation and combustion reaction, which destroys the native mineral structure and leads to the said inferior mechanical properties of the splinter material obtained by this method. In all the burning studies, the procedure focused only on the combustion of organic substances, and subsequent additional stabilisation of the remaining mineral substance was neglected (Mittelmeier).

The penetration of endogenous blood vessels into implants of inorganic cortical structures, such as those performed by Bassett et al. (1962), is next to impossible. Residual untreated autogenic cortical structures interfere with the remodelling process and are often only incorporated as dead foreign material.

For the sake of completeness, we also have to include in this discussion of natural calcium phosphates the tests performed more recently with mineral structures from corals. Roy and Linnehan (1974) used corals and starfish vertebrae, which contain aragonite and calcite, respectively, as starting materials for the preparation of apatite and whitlockite. By heat and pressure treatment with addition of ammonium phosphate and water, they produced hydroxyapatite and tricalcium phosphate, respectively, as well as whitlockite structures from the coral aragonite and the starfish calcite, while preserving the spatial structure of the original materials.

Holmes (1979) also produced hydroxyapatite from corals, and implanted it in jaw defects in dogs. After 12 months, he observed resorption of the implants in 29% of cases; after 2 months 11%, after 4 months 46%, and after 6 months 88% of the remaining implant surface had been filled with regenerated bone. Patel (1982) worked with Madreporaria (stone corals), which are largely composed of calcium carbonate with the crystal structure of aragonite, and performed preliminary animal experiments and clinical implants. Attempts to produce bone-replacement materials from coral substances have probably not been pursued further because of the availability of synthetically produced hydroxyapatites. Moreover, the use of calcium carbonate does not look very promising when compared with hydroxyapatite. We therefore decided not to include coral implants in our own experiments.

4.8 Pure Mineral Bone Pyrost

Collapat is not structurally stabile, in spite of its excellent bone-regeneration effect. Because many indications require a structurally stable osteoregenerative bone replacement, the development of such an implant material seemed desirable. In Mittelmeier's opinion, pure mineral bone, from which all organic matter had been totally removed, would probably be the most suitable structurally stable bone-replacement material, because its bone structures had developed in accordance with biomechanical principles and because of the natural mineral substance it contains. It was to be expected that natural mineral substance, which consists of up to 90% hydroxyapatite, would probably have the same osteoregenerative effect as was synthetic hydroxyapatite, against which no immunogenic interference arises, due to its total deproteination.

For these reasons, Mittelmeier took a renewed interest in the procedures for burning the organic substances in natural bone. However, he wished to avoid the mistakes that had led to the failure of "maceration by burning" in previous procedures. He developed a method which avoided the pitfalls of earlier burning procedures by eliminating prior storage in the frozen state (which causes bursting of the mineral structure due to freezing). Instead, premaceration was performed on the bone soft-tissue substances, and very gentle burning conditions, with only a low water vapour and gas pressure were chosen. With this procedure, it was possible to achieve complete disorganisation of the bone, without destroying the native crystal arrangement and bone structure. The resulting material was treated using a special sintering process, whereby the mineral particles were melted together to form a ceramic material, resulting in better-developed crystalline structures. Due to the gentle processing conditions, the bone tissue survives the critical burning phase without disintegrating into ashes (as was the case with earlier materials) while retaining its native structural features, and is then stabilised again by the sintering process. The bone basically retains its earlier shape. In comparison to native bone, the removal of all organic substances only causes shrinkage of the trabeculae, and therefore leads to a relative widening of the gaps between the meshes and to a slight general shrinkage of the preparation, which is of no consequence.

The gaps between the meshes are also relatively larger than in a bone splinter with the same original structure that has been treated only by soft-tissue maceration according to the procedure for the Kiel bone splinter. The gaps are also considerably larger than in most synthetic porous apatite and tricalcium-phosphate ceramic materials that have been investigated. This represents a considerable advantage, since material obtained by pyrolysis (burning) and sintering is much more amenable to rapid and complete penetration by granuloma tissue than are non-macerated bone transplants (e.g. spongiosa from a bone bank) or partly macerated bone (e.g. Kiel splinters). Therefore, for this material, one of Schweiberer's (1970) principal objections to Kiel bone splinters has been overcome, namely that the relatively broad fans of spongiosa "obstruct the path" of the penetrating granuloma tissue like a barrier. In this respect, this type of mineral bone also seems superior to ceramic materials made of synthetic porous hydroxyapatite, in which, due to the usual foaming process, the bubbly fan walls are often still present, and hinder the invasion of granuloma tissue deep into the material, so that the bone mostly unites only on the surface, and the implant is not completely penetrated or replaced. The mineral substance prepared by this method was named Pyrost, by analogy with the essential processing step of total disorganisation by pyrolysis.

A significant difference between Collapat and Pyrost is that Pyrost has sufficient structural stability for practical transplant purposes, even though it is a spongy substance. Of course, during the sintering process, the excellent tensile strength of natural bone – a collagen-fibre-composite material – is not attained. The tensile strength is also lower than that of the (partially) macerated Kiel splinter, which still contains collagen in the matrix and is, therefore, not very useful for immunological reasons.

Stability measurements in our biomechanics laboratory (Hopf and Hanser, personal communication) have shown that Pyrost has about 50% of the compressive strength of Kieler bone-splinter material, which is sufficient for practical transplant uses that require dimensional stability. Cortico-cancellous autografts do not have a high load tolerance, but only dimensional stability. In cases where a free defect has to be bridged, they always have to be protected by stable internal fixation or plaster. With this in mind, the limited stability of Pyrost is not really a practical disadvantage.

Pyrost is generally made from animal bones of the desired structure. In general, strips of easily accessible spongiosa several centimetres long and with a cross-section of 5 × 5 mm are recommended for this purpose. In principle, it is also possible to obtain cortico-spongy material through the Pyrost process. It is also possible to prepare entire bones as Pyrost, particularly bones of human origin.

Chemical analysis has confirmed that Pyrost no longer contains any organic material. Also, only trace carbon residues remain (Zitter 1983, personal communication).

X-ray crystallographic investigations have shown that Pyrost is about 93% hydroxy-apatite (natural bone is 90%), the rest being made up of about 7% alpha-tricalcium phosphate [Esper 1984, personal communication].

The following inorganic components were detected by spectroscopic analysis (atom-absorption spectroscopy):

1.	Main components:	Ca (38.4%) and P (18.9%)
2.	By-products:	(> 1%) Mg
3.	Small fractions:	(1%–0.1%) Cu
4.	Clear traces:	(< 0.1%) Sr, B, Ph, Bi
5.	Small traces:	(approx. 0.01%) Al, Ba, Si
6.	Rest:	O and H

Compared with the synthetic hydroxyapatite used in Collapat, more trace elements are present. These can also be detected in untreated natural bone. It seems particularly noteworthy that no iron, sodium, or potassium was detected in Pyrost.

Our own animal experiments confirmed the expected rapid penetration of the implant with granuloma tissue and the intensive osteoregeneration, both on the surface and in the gaps between the meshes. Following these favourable results, Pyrost has been subjected to clinical trial since 1983. To date, 350 patients who received Pyrost implants as treatment of pathological and operative bone defects have been studied (Fig. 4.2).

In view of the existing clinical experience, the excellent X-ray contrast of Pyrost is notable, particularly when compared with Collapat. This allows very good assessment of the progressing integration. We would like to mention here that very good bone regeneration has generally been observed in the implant area, and that no negative effects whatever, either general or local, have been observed.

Unlike Collapat, Pyrost does not have a local haemostyptic effect. Because of the ease with which Collapat can be modelled and its haemostyptic effect on the one hand, and the dimensional stability of Pyrost on the other, there are some preferred uses for each material in spite of overlapping indications. If relatively large, bleeding bone wounds have to be filled and bone regeneration is sought, then Collapat is to be preferred. If emphasis lies on the structural stabilisation of defects, then Pyrost is the better choice.

Collapat and Pyrost can also be used advantageously in combination, the bleeding bone defect being first covered with Collapt and then filled with Pyrost until the desired

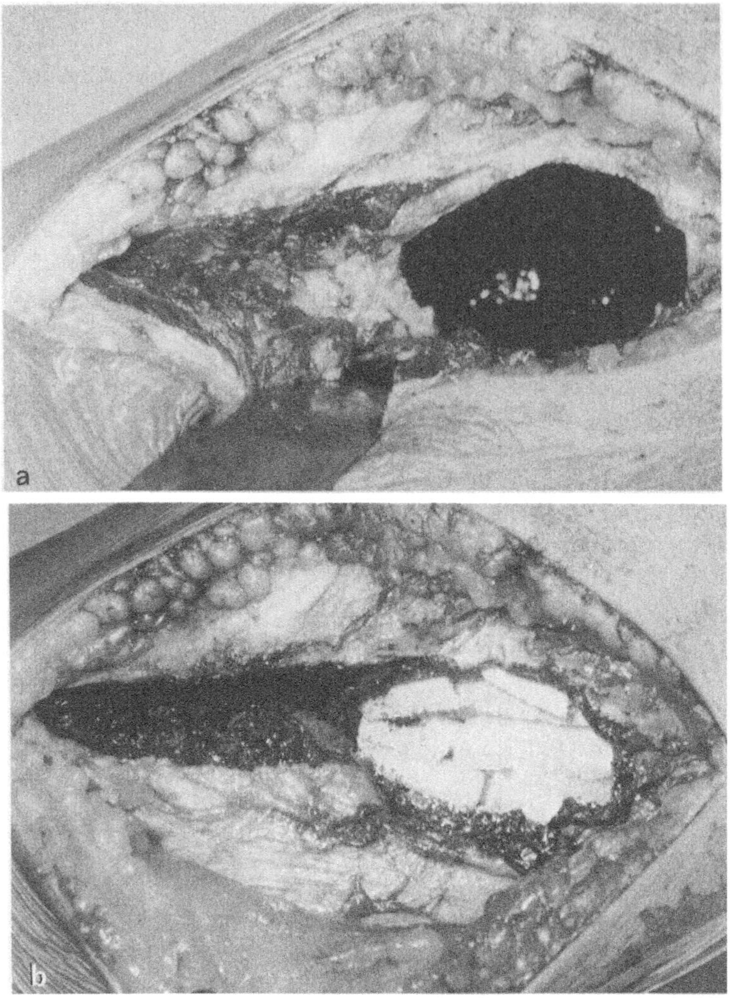

Fig. 4.2 a, b. Clinical aspect of Pyrost implants. **a** Excision of a tumour in the head of the tibia (large giant-cell tumour). **b** Filling with Pyrost trabeculae. The implant is dimensionally stable and promotes bone regeneration

shape of the bone is obtained, possibly followed by another layer of Collapat. (In the clinical studies we have performed so far, however, we have tended to use either one or the other material, in order to test the specific effect of each material.)

Pyrost was first publicly described at the German Congress for Plastic and Reconstructive Surgery in 1983 (Katthagen and Mittelmeier 1983b). In 1984 (Mittelmeier and Katthagen 1984) we discussed in particular the "new approaches in bone replacement" which had become possible with Collapat and Pyrost.

5 Experimental Section

5.1 Test Animals and Animal Housing

Bastard rabbits obtained from local breeders were used as test animals irrespective of their strain or sex. The rabbits had an average weight of 3.14 kg. They were delivered to the laboratory not later than 1 week before the start of the test, and acclimatised to the housing conditions and the feed. The animals were kept in single UNO metal cages (model B 3/3, type K) at 22°C and 50% relative humidity in natural daylight with a day-night rhythm. A standard dry-feed diet which contained 16.5% raw protein, 13.5% raw fibre, 1.2% calcium, 0.65% phosphorus, 10000 IU vitamin A and 2000 IU vitamin D_3 per kg of feed mixture was given. The animals were offered standard tap water ad libitum.

5.2 Operating Method

The operations were carried out in a conventional operating theatre with the animals lying supine on an operating table. They were anaesthetized using a mask and a semi-open system. During the induction phase of the anaesthesia the rabbits received 3.5–4 vol% of halothane, thereafter 2.5 vol%. Also, 1 l oxygen and 2 l NO per minute were administered (Fig. 5.1).

After shaving, disinfection and sterile draping of the operation site, the femoral condyles were exposed by means of a medial longitudinal incision. Initially, a substance defect was created by means of a 3.2 mm drill and was subsequently expanded with a 6 mm drill. All the drill holes were carefully rinsed with Ringer's solution and cleaned out, so that any abraded particles formed during drilling were removed. These defects were then completely filled with the corresponding implant material, or left open in the case of control cavities. The wound was sutured atraumatically in two layers with 3.0 Vicryl and Prolene. After final disinfection an adhesive spray bandage was applied to the operation area (Fig. 5.2).

This operating technique was recommended by Mittelmeier (personal communication) and had already been used successfully in experimental studies by Nizard (1981). Maatz et al. (1954) had first described the "spongiosa test" and produced a 5 mm substance defect in the dog. Schweiberer (1970) had also carried out experiments with the spongiosa test in the dog (Fig. 5.3).

As with any experimental investigation, and particularly in animal testing, the validity of the experimental model for the question being researched is of decisive importance for the evaluation of the test results. For this reason we wish to introduce the model which we chose here without going into the details of the experimental results at this stage. In order to be able to study the stimulating effect on bone regeneration of varios implantation materials, the investigations naturally have to be performed on an animal model. In

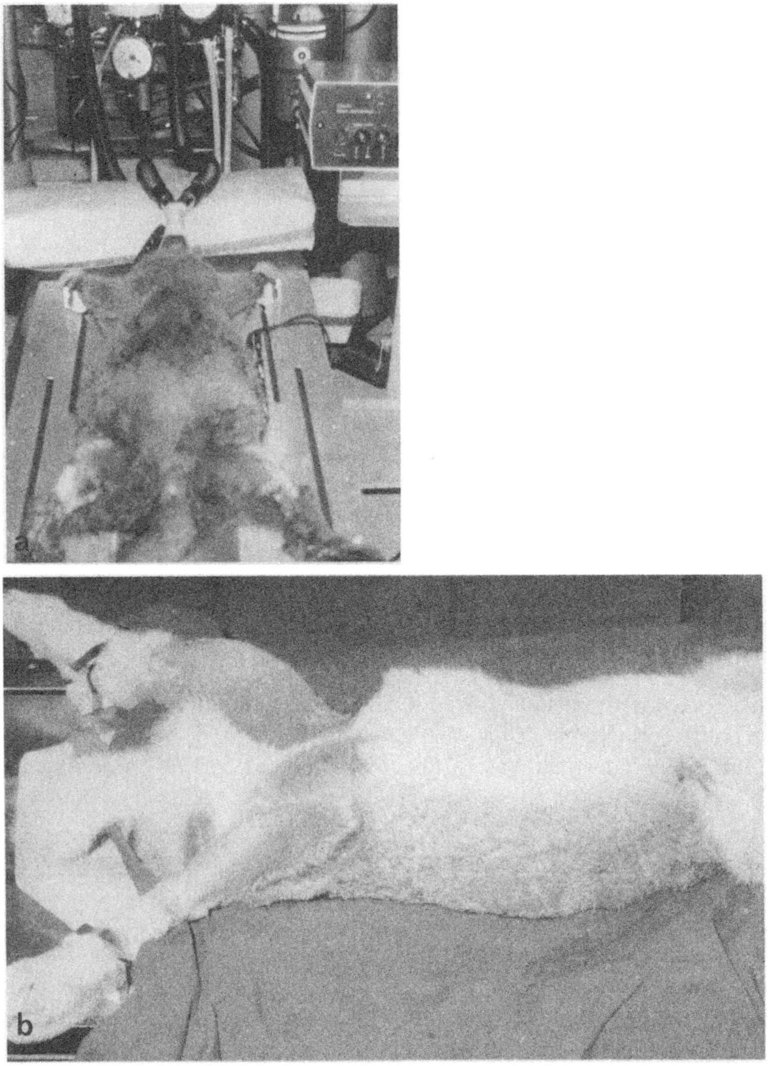

Fig. 5.1a, b. Position of the rabbit on the operating table. The anaesthesia apparatus is shown in the *background*

accordance with the requirements of the law on the protection of animals, animal experiments should, as far as possible, be performed on lower animals. Because of the small dimensions of their bones, mice or rats are only partially suitable for the purpose of this project.

Since the scope of this work includes serial investigations of ten different implant materials and a total of 96 experimental animals were needed, large animals such as monkeys, sheep, pigs or dogs did not come into consideration for cost reasons. At a cost of 1500 DM per dog (and this is a modest estimate), the purchase price and the housing

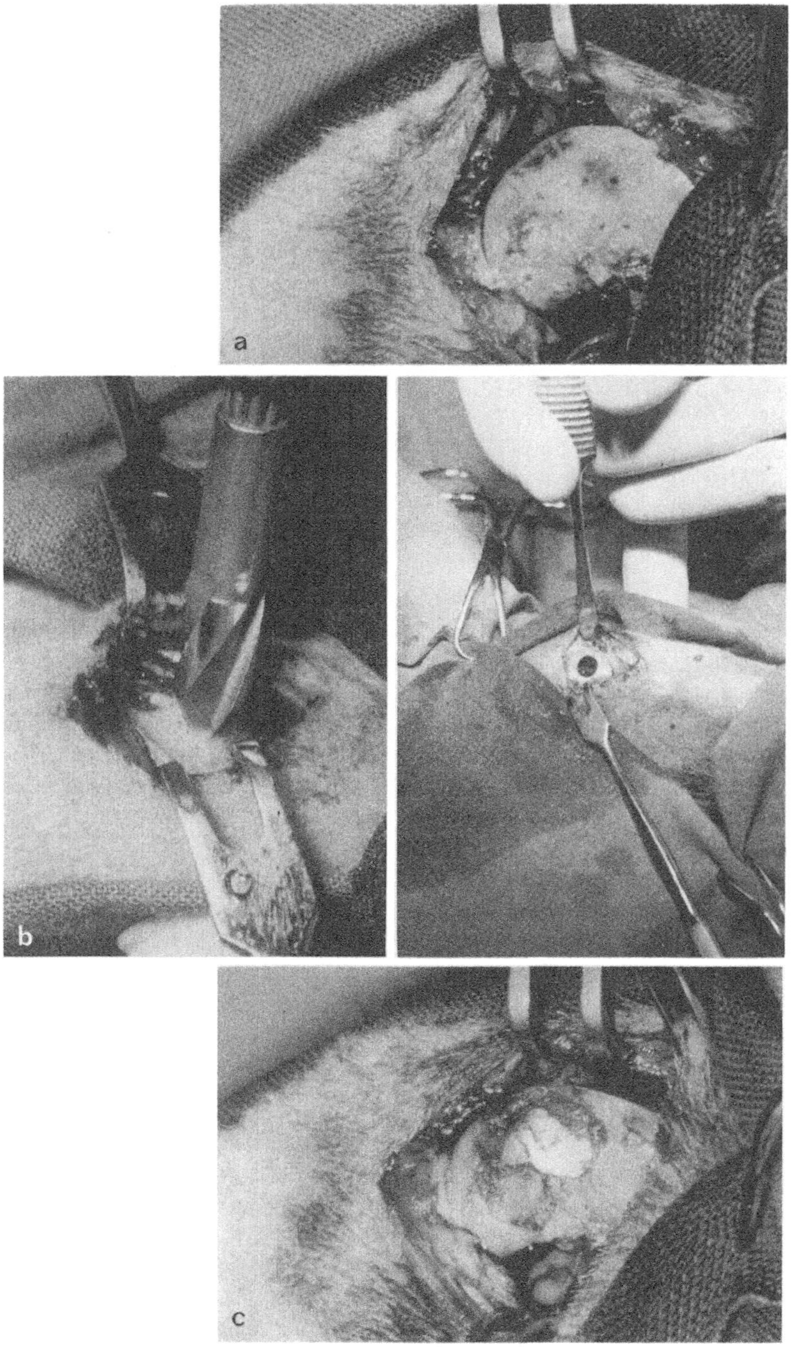

Fig. 5.2. **a** Exposure of the femoral condyle. **b** Drilling with 6 mm drill. **c** Cavity before and after filling with Collapat E

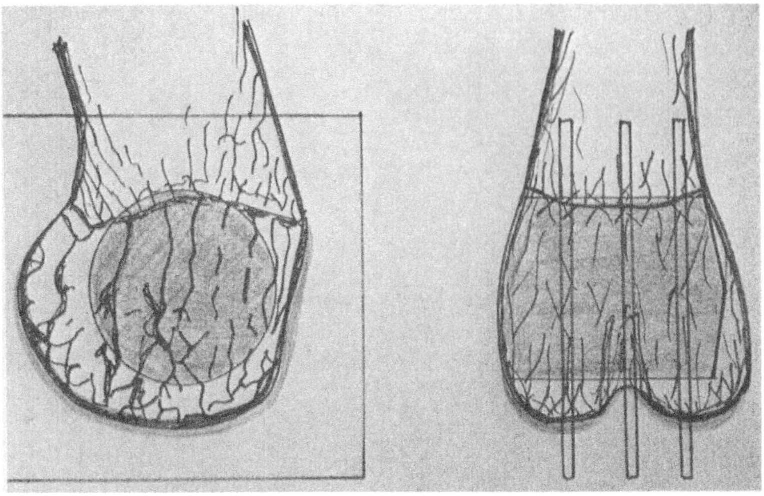

Fig. 5.3. Cavity test. Schematic representation of the drilled cavity (*left*) and the section plane of the histological preparations (*right*)

cost alone for the animals required for the serial investigations would amount to approximately 200000 DM. Because of the lower purchase price and easier housing, the rabbit was the preferred test animal.

It may be said, and this objection is partly justified, that regeneration tests on rabbit bones give results which are too favourable due to the excellent bone-regeneration capacity of the rabbit. Along this line, A. Hopf argued at an orthopaedic congress in 1957 that:

"Experiments on rabbits cannot be taken as evidence for man. This is an experience which has been quoted already for the past 10 years in every publication dealing with experimental work on bones and which we should consider as binding also today. The rabbit has quite an excellent callous-forming capacity. You only have to inject 1 cm^3 of alcohol into the muscles of a rabbit and this will lead to the formation of bone, as has been observed by several authors. The spongiosa test is misleading in a scientific evaluation. To use it as the basis of a clinical study only because even the worst bone tissue demonstrates an excellent activity in this test, entirely due to the recipient bed, would not be acceptable. It is, therefore, not surprising that even now in the spongiosa test, in agreement with the investigations of Maatz as well as with our own, the macerated bone tissue shows excellent results, even better results than the autoplastic one."

With regard to the test animal it must, however, be pointed out that the bone-regeneration capacity of the dog, at least in the spongiosa test, is no worse than that of the rabbit. The experimental investigations by Schweiberer demonstrate that, for defects of 5 mm diameter, there is often complete bone reconstruction in the defect after 14–15 days, entirely due to the recipient bed. For this reason, Schweiberer (1970) chose a larger diameter of 10 mm for some of his test animals. However, his illustrated series of ten spongiosa defects of 10 mm diameter show that, even in this case, the empty cavity was soon filled with regenerated bone. The defect cavities were almost completely filled spontaneously with regenerated bone after 17, 20 and 20 days. For this reason, Ecke (1967, 1976) suggested carrying out bone-regeneration tests using the so-called *compact test* on the diaphysis, because this is also the site of most clinical applications.

In our opinion, however, the regenerative capacity of the spongy recipient bed is also limited, and always depends on the size of the defect in relation to the chosen bone section. It is certainly not possible to compare a 6 mm substance defect in the rabbit with an equally large defect in the dog, since much greater relative damage is caused by a 6 mm defect – also with regard to blood circulation – in the rabbit than in the dog. It is a well-known fact from clinical experience that smaller bone defects can be closed, also in man, purely by the regenerative capacity of the remaining bone tissue, but that this is no longer possible in defects above a certain size. As can be seen from the investigations by Schweiberer (1970), even a 10 mm substance defect in the dog is still too small, since it is spontaneously and completely overgrown after only 3 weeks. A 6 mm substance defect in the rabbit femoral condyle is barely feasible and destroys approximately half of the femoral condyle, which on average has a size of 1–1.5 cm. In addition, when the defect is achieved by a machine-driven, gross structured drill head (Fig. 5.2b), parts of the surrounding bone are destroyed, too. Such a large bone defect would not be possible in the region of the diaphysis, because it would cause a fracture, which in turn would initiate a regeneration process. Also, a stabilising osteosynthesis would be required at the same time. We have, however, taken the previously mentioned criticisms of bone-regeneration studies in the rabbit into consideration, and have performed a large series of control experiments. We are therefore in a position to evaluate implant-induced bone regeneration in comparison with spontaneous formation of new bone. Based on the results of these control experiments, it can be shown that **the chosen experimental model is valid in spite of all the critical comments regarding the large size of the defect in relation to the size of the bone,** and is thus suitable, from the view-points of animal welfare, cost and easy animal housing, **for comparative serial investigations of different implantation materials in beds with strong regenerative capacity.**

5.3 Histological Technique

5.3.1 General Aspects of Undecalcified Bone Histology

The principal advantages of the *undecalcified* histological preparation of bone specimens are mentioned below:

1. Less shrinkage of the tissue specimens
2. The preservation of minerals as essential constituents of the bone
3. Better differentiation of mineralised and non-mineralised bone structures
4. Better conservation of soft-tissue structures and their relative positions by elimination of decalcifying acids during the preparation
5. The possibility for microradiographic investigation
6. The possibility of following the process of new-bone formation and bone reconstruction by polychrome fluorescent staining of the histological preparation
7. The possibility of investigating hard implants (in this study, mineral-based bone-replacement materials such as apatite and calcium-phosphate ceramics), with their adjacent tissue structures, in thin sections

There are also *disadvantages* associated with the undecalcified preparation technique. The unfavourable effect of the polymerisation heat on the tissue specimens must be mentioned primarily, but also considerable time is required and the high cost of preparation.

Expertise in undecalcified bone histology is still not widespread today. General procedures are described in various publications, but they in themselves are not sufficient for successful application of the undecalcified-bone-histology technique. We would therefore like to give a detailed description of the histological technique used in this study, and to give an overview of the published literature on this subject. Our intention is to introduce other research groups who do not yet have practical experience with the technique to undecalcified bone histology and its histomorphometric evaluation (Katthagen and Bechtel 1985).

The introduction of polymer embedding was a prerequisite for the preparation of undecalcified bone sections. Puckett (1941) described the use of *methacrylate* as an embedding material. Roofe et al. (1949) developed a *microtome saw* for the preparation of 20–30 μm thin bone sections. The loss of material per section with this microtome was approximately 150 μm. They used so-called bioplastic as the embedding material. Kropp (1954) described a method for accelerating the polymer-embedding process by using a technique which is common in metallurgy, namely performing the polymerisation at 130 °C under pressure. This technique, however, could only be applied to samples with a thickness greater than 2 mm.

For the preparation of acceptably thin sections, embedding in pure methacrylate proved far too difficult. Boellaard and von Hirsch (1959) were able to make sections as thin as 3 μm by the addition of a plasticiser (polyethylene glycol). They adapted the method, which had initially been developed for investigation of brain specimens, to the preparation of histological sections from undecalcified bone specimens (Hirsch and Boellaard 1958). The present technique of embedding in methylmethacrylate essentially originates from this work. A comprehensive historical survey of the development of plastic embedding and a precise description of the technique can be found in the work of Schenk (1965) on the histological preparation of undecalcified bone specimens. The entire histological preparation method, including the techniques of fixation, dehydration, impregnation, embedding, cutting, posttreatment and staining was further improved by Burkhardt (1966a, b). Detailed descriptions of the preparation were presented by Henschke and Pesch (1978), Eisen (1979) and Schönfeldt and Bössmann (1980).

Since the polymerisation heat generated during the polymer-embedding process considerably impairs or even prevents the histochemical assessment of methacrylate-embedded bone sections, Westen et al. (1981) have modified the methacrylate-embedding technique so that it can be performed at temperatures as low as 20 °C.

5.3.2 Polychrome Fluorescent Staining

Polymer embedding attained particular significance through the discovery of *fluorescent microscopic intra-vital staining* with tetracycline (Milch et al. 1958; Harris 1960; Harris et al. 1962, 1968; Frost 1961; Eger et al. 1964).

Olerud and Lorenzi (1970) introduced *polychrome fluorescent staining,* which allowed dynamic representation of bone changes by means of bone sections. Rahn summarised the possibilities offered by *polychromic sequence labelling* in 1976. In this technique, the following intravital colourants are injected into animals at *defined time intervals* during the experiment:

1. Achromycin yellow: 10–15 mg/kg body weight
2. Calcein green: 10–20 mg/kg body weight
3. Xylenol orange: 60–90 mg/kg body weight
4. Alizarin complex red: 20–30 mg/kg body weight

According to our experience with rabbits a single *subcutaneous* administration is sufficient for achromycin yellow and calcein green but not for xylenol orange or alizarin complex red. The latter are not incorporated sufficiently upon subcutaneous administration, and are eclipsed when evaluated together with achromycin yellow and calcein green. They should, therefore, be administered to the rabbit intravenously and at higher dosages.

5.3.3 Fixation and Embedding of the Bone Specimens

The excised bone specimens, from which any remaining soft tissue has been removed, are fixed in 40% *methanol* for 24 h. A longer fixation period is not detrimental to further processing. For the polymer embedding to be successful, the embedding material must be able to penetrate the bone specimen completely. This requires thorough *dehydration* and *lipid extraction* of the fixed bone specimens, performed in an *graded alcohol* series, for 24 h in each solution, according to the following scheme:

1. Ethanol 80%
2. Ethanol 96%
3. Ethanol 100%
4. Ethanol 100% + acetone (1:1)
5. Acetone
6. Ethanol 100% + acetone (1:1)
7. Ethanol

Incomplete lipid removal can disturb the polymerisation process; residual acetone in the bone may lead to bubble formation.

The *embedding* of the fixed, dehydrated and de-fatted bone specimen is performed in various stages with the following solutions:

1. Methylmethacrylate solution I (monomeric methylmethacrylate)
2. Methylmethacrylate solution II (100 ml methylmethacrylate + 2 mg benzoyl peroxide)
3. Methylmethacrylate solution III (100 ml methylmethacrylate + 4 g benzoyl peroxide + 25 ml plastoid N).

Benzoyl peroxide is used as a polymerisation catalyst. It is explosive when in the dry state, and therefore contains 30% added water. Before use it is dried in an oven at 37 °C.

Plastoid N (nanylphenolpolyglycolether acetate) is a plasticiser which makes it possible to cut sections from the block. Plastoid N is water soluble and miscible in any ratio with methylmethacrylate.

Work with methylmethacrylate should always be performed under an exhaust hood, since it can sensitise the skin, and is an irritant to the eyes and the respiratory system. The actual embedding procedure is as follows:

Flat-bottomed flasks, which are first pre-polymerised, are used as *embedding moulds*. For this purpose they are filled with 10 ml methylmethacrylate solution III, and evacuated in an exsiccator by means of a water-jet pump. (We always keep a number of pre-polymerised embedding moulds in stock, in order to save time.) The pre-polymerisation period is approx. 2–3 days, and the temperature is initially set to 40°C and then increased by 2°–3°C each day. By this procedure one obtains a methylmethacrylate carrier on the bottom for further embedding. To remove the polymerisation heat, the flat-bottomed flasks are placed in a water bath, whose level is approximately the same as the methylmethacrylate level in the flasks. The flat-bottomed flasks are lightly covered, but not sealed airtight, to avoid the condensation of droplets on the side or the stopper, which could lead to the formation of bubbles. If a few *air bubbles* do not interfere with further processing, the flasks can also be closed airtight. This accelerates the polymerisation.

The bone specimens to be embedded are then transferred into non-prepolymerised flat bottomed flasks, and covered with monomeric methylmethacrylate (solution I). These flat-bottomed flasks are placed in an exsiccator and evacuated for about 24 h. On the following day, the monomeric methylmethacrylate solution is discarded (not into the sink) and the bone specimens together with the labels are transferred into other non-prepolymerised flat-bottomed flasks. These are then filled with methylmethacrylate solution II, and are again evacuated for 24 h. On the 3rd day, the methylmethacrylate mixture II is again discarded, and the side of the bone which is to be sectioned is pressed into the pre-polymerised bottom of the prepared flat-bottomed flask.

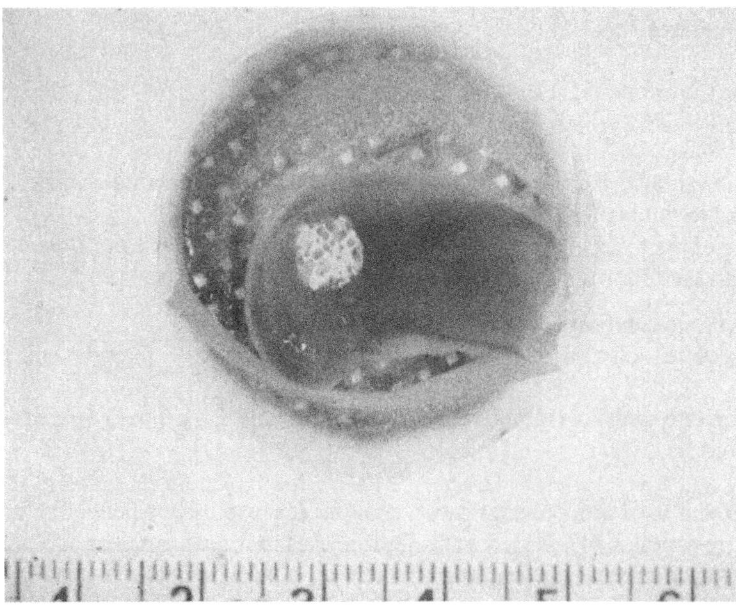

Fig. 5.4. Embedding of the samples in methylmethacrylate, shown here after filling with Pyrost

The labels, which are marked with pencil, should be fixed on the inner side of the flasks, so that they can later be read easily. Finally, the methylmethacrylate solution III is carefully added in such a way that the bone is not washed off, and remains in the predetermined position required for the subsequent cutting procedure. The polymerisation then takes place under the same conditions as described above for the prepolymerisation, except that initially a lower temperature of 35 °C is used. A certain loss from evaporation has to be taken into consideration, and the initial methylmethacrylate level should therefore be 2–3 cm higher than the bone.

The embedding procedure is complete after 8–10 days. The totally polymerised flasks are then wrapped in cellulose, and smashed with a hammer to release the *methylmethacrylate blocks*. The top layer of the block often does not polymerise completely, and is cut off with a band saw (Fig. 5.4).

The completely polymerised blocks can now be fixed in the section cutter according to the instructions. For section cutting we used the Leitz *sawing microtome* to prepare 70 μm-thick sections which can be examined directly by microradiography and fluorescence microscopy without further processing.

5.3.4 Microradiography

The microradiography technique used involves the *X-ray representation of thin 70 μm sections or ground sections of undecalcified bone preparations*. The exposed film negatives are examined under the microscope. The technique of microradiography goes back to Clark (1931). It was subsequently further developed for the quantitative investigation of bone tissue by Engstroem (1946), Holmstrand (1957), Gück (1957) and Jowsey et al. (1965).

The microradiographic investigation of our own preparations was performed according to the contact microradiographic method described by Freitag and Ruppersberg (1972) and Freitag and Stetter (1973) at the oral surgery clinic of the University of Homburg/Saar. In order to obtain maximal resolution, the distance between the object and the film is kept as small as possible. To achieve this, the preparation is placed into a cassette and pressed directly onto the film with the help of a foil, and a negative pressure of 3 torr is created in the cassette by means of an air-suction pump (Leybold-Heraeus). The investigations were carried out with a spectrometer tube (AGTI 61), an X-ray generator (Kristalloflex 700) and an adjustable transformer (Siemens). The X-rays generated in the spectrometer tube were passed through a titanium filter and an evacuated chamber at 65 torr. The focusfilm distance was 25 cm. For negatives with maximum resolution and contrast, the corresponding film material is required. We used Kodak Spectroscopic Film 50-616, type 649-GH. The exposure time was 14–16 min at 10 mV and 50 mA. The films exposed in this manner were developed with Kodak Developer D-19.

5.3.5 Fluorescence Microscopy

For optimum excitation of the various fluorochromes, the excitation and emission wavelengths must be known. Rahn determined the wavelengths of the excitation and emission maxima of a series of bone fluorochromes in his thesis (Table 5.1).

Table 5.1. Wavelengths of the excitation and emission maxima for different bone fluorochromes

Substance	Excitation in apatite (nm)	Emission in bone (nm)
Calcein blue	350	445
Xylenol orange	377	615
Calcein	495	540
Alizarin complex one	580	625
Oxytetracycline	425	525

In fluorescence microscopy, both the *reflection* and the *transillumination* techniques can be used. In the transillumination technique, some of the light is absorbed by the preparation, and the light intensity, which is already weak, is thereby further reduced. We therefore limited ourselves to reflection fluorescence. With this method – as we pointed out earlier – the microtome sections of 50–70 μm thickness can be used directly, without further processing. They are simply glued onto the slide with Entellan. For observation and photographic documentation, we used the Zeiss photomicroscope with a fluorescence facility. It is equipped with an HBO 50 mercury lamp. This equipment is not suitable for making survey pictures, but is well suited for observation with 20-fold magnification and above. The best visibility of the individual fluorochromes is obtained with specially adapted band-pass filters with only very narrow transmission ranges. For the simultaneous observation of all fluorochromes, it is necessary to excite in the UV range, and the rejector filter should ideally transmit the entire spectrum of fluorescence emission. Special filter combinations are available for this purpose: excitation filter BP 365, partition mirror FT 390 and rejector filter LP 390 (Rahn 1976). Because of the low light intensity of the fluorescence, the use of high sensitivity films is recommended for photographic documentation.

5.3.6 Refinement of the Sectioning Technique

For light microscopy it is necessary to prepare microsections of 3–5 μm thickness. Before cutting the sections, the methylmethacrylate block should be adjusted with a small bow-saw in such a way that a small residue of methylmethacrylate remains attached to the bone. After fastening the block, the slide should carefully be moved into the vicinity of the knife. The knives and the block should be covered with cutting fluid (from WIV).

We used the K-Microtome from Jung as our cutting instrument. For bone histology, special *hard-sectioning microtome knives* are required. These are expensive, and they rapidly become blunt. The initial sections are therefore made with a blunt knife in order to save the sharp knives for the final sections.

The microsections are lifted off with a pair of fine tweezers, and placed on a slide coated with *chromium-alum gelatin.* With the help of a small brush and with *diluent solution* (30 ml butylglycol from WIV + 70 ml 70% ethanol), the sections are brushed until any *wrinkles* which may be present have been smoothed out completely. This procedure is carried out under a magnifying glass. One then takes a Kisol film which has already been cut to match the size of the slide and places it on the section. The excess diluent fluid is wiped off with soft paper (e.g. paper handkerchief). The sections are then fastened in a *slide press* or a screw clamp and stored in an incubator at 56°C overnight.

The *preparation of the chromium-alum-gelatin solution* is as follows: 4.5 g gelatin is first dissolved at 75°C in 1 l distilled water. A 4% chromium-alum solution is then prepared, and 1 l filtered gelatin solution is mixed with 38.5 ml chromium-alum solution. Two drops of Pril detergent are added to the mixture.

The slides are coated with chromium-alum gelatin by a detailed procedure. First the slides are stored in 2% HCl solution for at least 30 min, and then washed with distilled water. They are then neutralised with 2% NaOH solution for 2 min, and again washed with water. Then, they are placed in the oven for drying. Following this, the slides are immersed in the previously described chromium-alum-gelatin solution for 2 min. They are then rotated in air with in a special basket until the chromium-alum-gelatin layer has dried. Following this, the slides are stored at 56°C in the incubator until they are used.

The *adhesion of the section* on the slide coated with chromium-alum gelatin is increased by the incubation at 56°C. This is very important, since a great risk exists that the sections may float away during subsequent deplastification and staining.

Deplastification is performed with the help of 2-methoxyethyl acetate. Three staining cuvettes are filled with 2-methoxyethyl acetate. (Since the 2-methoxyethyl acetate is used up very rapidly, it is advisable to renew it for each deplastification.) The slides coated with the sections are immersed for 10 min in each of the three staining cuvettes containing 2-methoxyethyl acetate. The deplastification step is followed by treatment in a decreasing-ethanol series graded down to distilled water:

1. Ethanol 100% for 5 min
2. Ethanol 96% for 5 min
3. Ethanol 80% for 5 min
4. Ethanol 70% for 5 min
5. Distilled water

5.3.7 Staining of Undecalcified Bone Preparations

We used mainly the Masson-Goldner and the Giemsa staining techniques. Although corresponding staining procedures can be found in the older textbooks on histological techniques (Romeis 1968; Burkhardt 1966a, b) they are not applicable to bone histology without modification.

5.3.7.1 Masson-Goldner (MG) Staining

Iron haematoxylin, ponceau de xylidine, phosphotungstic acid, orange G and light green were used as staining solutions. After deplastification, the sections fixed on the slides were treated with iron-haematoxylin solution for 15 min. Thereafter the slides were rinsed with tap water until no more colour was given off. The slides were then transferred into ponceau de xylidine. This solution consists of 2 g ponceau, 1 g acid fuchsin, 0.4 ml glacial acetic acid and 200 ml distilled water. The preparations are then rinsed two or three times in water and then in 1% acetic acid. Next follows 7-min staining with phosphotungstic acid orange G. This solution is prepared with 2 g phosphotungstic acid

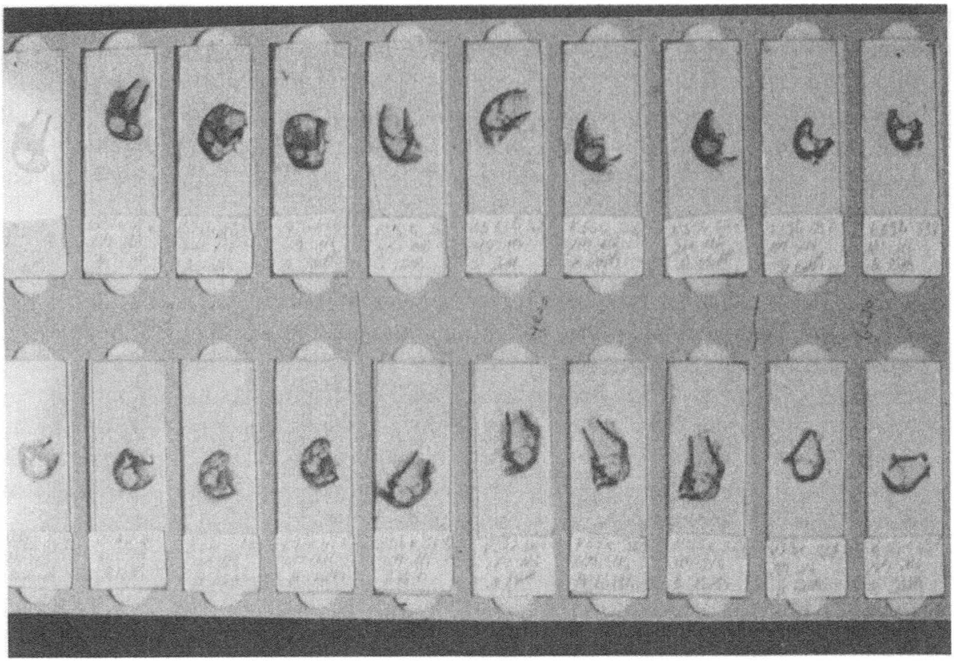

Fig. 5.5. Microsections of 5 µm after Masson-Goldner (MG) staining. The drilled cavity defect is clearly visible macroscopically. A series of preparations with gelatin fillings is shown

and 1 g orange G in 200 ml distilled water. Then follows another rinse with water, then with 1% acetic acid. Finally, the slides are transferred into the light green solution for 15 min. This solution is made up of 0.4 g light green and 0.4 ml glacial acetic acid in 200 ml distilled water. After rinsing with water, 1% acetic acid and again with water, the preparations are immersed three times each in 70% and 100% ethanol solutions (Fig. 5.5).

5.3.7.2 Giemsa Staining

The deplastified preparations are transferred into freshly prepared Giemsa solution (40 ml Giemsa; Merck 9204 + 160 ml distilled water) for 30 min, and then immersed three times in 1% acetic acid solution. Following this, the preparations are immersed three to four times in 100% ethanol solution and then rinsed twice for 7 min each in isopropyl alcohol and then in xylene. The preparations stained in this manner are then covered with Entellan and dried.

5.3.8 Histomorphometry

Classical histology encompasses qualitative assessment of cells and tissues as well as alterations in cells and tissues. The scope of this work, which is a comparative assessment of the influence of different bone-replacement materials on bone regeneration, calls for a *quantitative assessment* of the amount of newly formed bone as a function of the corresponding implantation material and time. The quantitative comparison of bone regeneration under the influence of these materials, with spontaneous bone regeneration using the best transplantation material available – autogenous spongiosa – as a positive control, permits an exact assessment of the influence of the different materials on bone regeneration. An attempt to quantify this bone regeneration was made in earlier studies. Lentz (1955) used a circular *measuring eyepiece* and various concentrically delimited *measuring areas* to obtain a *semi-quantitative assessment.* This procedure was later adopted by Schweiberer (1970). Although this procedure yields more information than classical histology, it allows only a crude quantitative estimate, particularly of the bone distribution over the defect cavity, and does *not* constitute an *accurate* measurement of the bone which has actually grown.

Surface-area measurements have also been made using enlargements of photographs or drawings of the investigated tissues. Areas of the picture that represent individual structural elements are cut out and weighed, and the relative weights of the paper cuttings are used to calculate the corresponding relative surface areas. This procedure is still relatively imprecise, time-consuming and complicated, and is hardly applicable to the scope of our work, since the fine network of the regenerated bone can only be evaluated by cutting out a paper print with scissors when extreme magnifications are used.

The *dot-counting procedure* uses a *dot matrix,* which is projected onto the object's surface by the measuring eyepiece. The numbers of dots in the different structural elements are determined, and the relative surface areas calculated.

Considerable attention has been given to bone histomorphometry in the context of metabolic bone diseases. Merz (1967) and Merz and Schenk (1970) described the surface- and distance-measuring techniques known at the time, and rated the dot-counting procedure as the method of choice for surface-area determination. For volume determination, the authors used the *distance-measuring* technique with the help of semi-circular waves, and showed that under certain circumstances the surface area of the section and the perimeter lines of a histological preparation may be used to calculate *volume sizes* in a tissue specimen. By the combination of a dot matrix with these semi-circular waves, it is possible to measure the surface areas and the distances in a single operation, and to transform the data obtained into spatial, three-dimensional values. These techniques have been widely adopted for the quantitative determination of bone reconstruction and are still being used today (Schenk 1967; Schenk et al. 1969; Schenk and Merz 1969; Ellis and Peart 1972; Bordier and Tun Chot 1972; Delling 1974; Krempien et al. 1978; Melsen et al. 1978; Teitelbaum and Bates, 1980). For these investigations, undecalcified bone histology, which we also use, is a prerequisite, and the Masson-Goldner staining technique is normally used.

Further approaches to quantitative bone assessment are *microradiography* (Engstroem 1946; Holmstrand 1957; Jowsey et al. 1965) and *fluorescence microscopy* (Gelhard 1980; Rahn et al. 1980).

New developments in the field of quantitative tissue investigation have come from the possibilities offered by *micro-electronics* with semi-automatic and fully automatic systems. In *semi-automatic systems* the object to be evaluated is projected onto a measuring surface. The perimeters of the tissue structures are determined by following the contours with a measuring pen, whereby the electronic circuitry registers and adds up the perimeters of the corresponding surfaces. For this purpose, Leitz offers an *ASM analyser,* which Vernejoul et al. (1981) used in their bone histomorphometric investigations.

The possibility of using *automatic quantitative methods* has occasionally been mentioned recently (Siebert et al. 1976; Runge et al. 1979; Rahn et al. 1980). The *texture-analysis system* (TAS-Leitz) which we used initially allows automatic, computer-controlled quantitative evaluation of histological preparations, and is therefore well suited for image analysis, both in routine assessment of metabolic bone diseases and for experimental investigation of osteoregeneration in animals. We have previously described this quantitative method in experimental bone histology (Katthagen and Mittelmeier 1983a). In our investigations we used – as mentioned earlier – undecalcified bone sections of 5 μm thickness embedded in methylmethacrylate and stained according to Masson-Goldner, which permitted good evaluation both in the survey and also at the highest magnification level.

The pictures of these bone sections were taken directly through the Orthoplan microscope (Leitz), by a black and white television camera (Bosch), which is attached to a computer and can differentiate between various shades of grey. The contrast value of the trabeculae, which is already high in undecalcified bone sections with Masson-Goldner staining, can be further increased by the use of a *red filter.* This facilitates accurate calibration of the apparatus and accurate marking of the bone structures to be evaluated (Figs. 5.6 and 5.7).

In predetermined *electronic measuring sectors,* which can be chosen at will, the units of surface area occupied by a particular grey shade can be measured electronically at the

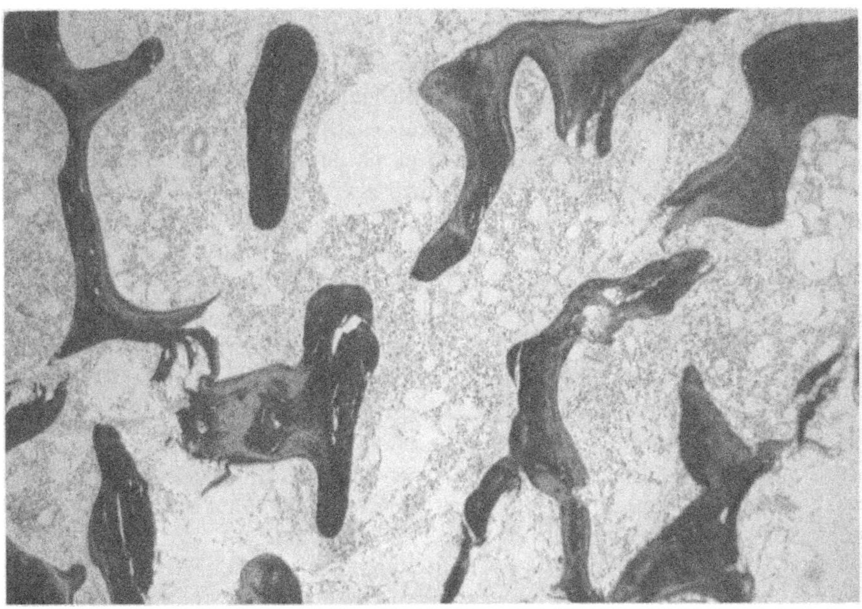

Fig. 5.6. Histological section 5 μm thick of human hip punch-biopsy. Mineralised bone (green in colour representation) and osteoid (red) cannot be differentiated in black and white representation. Masson-Goldner (MG)

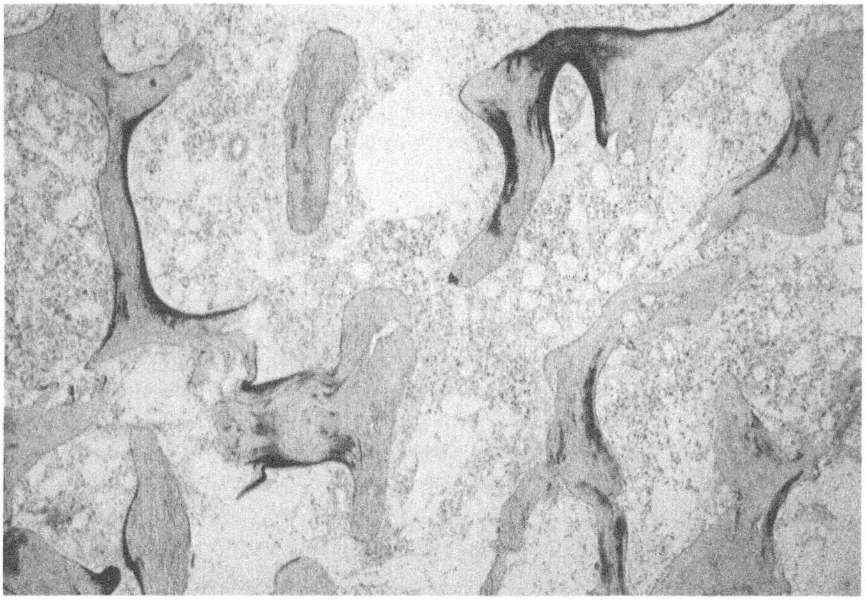

Fig. 5.7. Selective increase in contrast applied to the same preparation as in Fig. 5.6. By the use of green filters the mineralised (green) structures become paler and the non-mineralised red structures are emphasized. The same principle can be used to increase the contrast of mineralised structures with a red filter

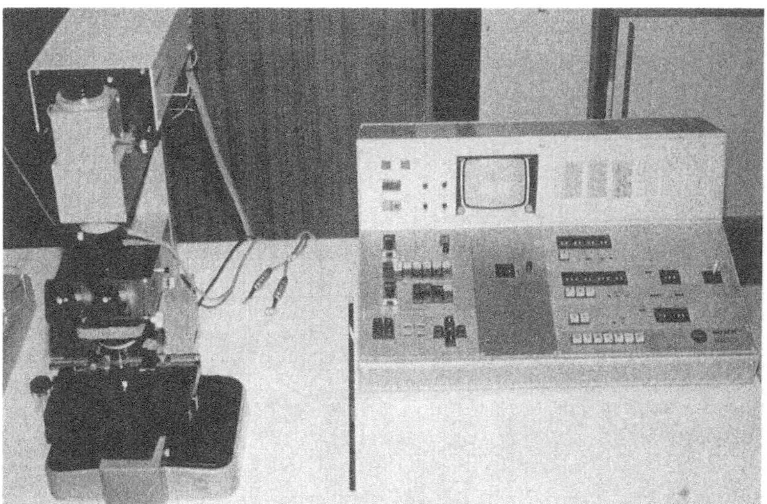

Fig. 5.8. Texture-analysis system (TAS-Leitz); *left,* microscope with television camera; *right,* console with control monitor

push of a button and later transformed into percentage (Fig. 5.8). Quantitative image analysis thus permits accurate objective assessment of the mineralised bone content of a microsection, expressed as a percentage.

There are, of course, also possibilities for error with this system. These arise from the shape and the position of the chosen measuring sector. The *transverse* bone defects that we drilled in the femoral condyles of the rabbit, with a diameter of 6 mm, ideally give a *circular* defect with a diameter of 6 mm upon longitudinal section. However, we could not always actually obtain a circular defect, because the axis of drilling and the section plane were *not* always *strictly perpendicular*.

If a cylinder is sectioned obliquely, an oval instead of a circular cross-section is obtained. Also, it is not possible to prevent the relatively large drill head from tearing particles of fine bone out of the tissue matrix beyond its circumference. The defect therefore becomes somewhat *irregular* and *larger* than 6 mm in diameter.

After an initial series of tests with the Leitz-TAS system, we carried out subsequent investigations, including the studies reported here, with the interactive image-analysis system (IBAS from Kontron). This system again projects the histological slide, by means of a microscope and a television camera, onto a television screen. In contrast to the TAS system it is, however, possible to mark the measuring sector accurately by defining its contour (Figs. 5.9–5.11).

The relative surface areas of the newly formed bone in the defect cavities were calculated. As a matter of principle, at least three different sections per test were evaluated. In one test series (Collapat E in comparison to an empty cavity), ten sections were evaluated per test to determine the variance of the test results. For this purpose, serial sections were made, and every 50 μm a section was selected and evaluated. The purpose of performing multiple determinations was to minimize the measuring error.

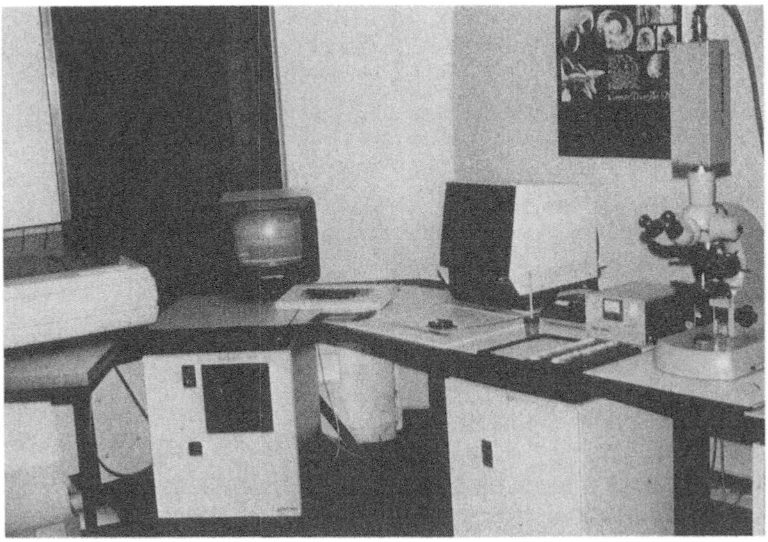

Fig. 5.9. Interactive image-analysis system (IBAS-Kontron; Duesseldorf FRG). From *left* to *right* are shown: printer, computer with keyboard and monitor, second monitor for image processing and microscope with television camera

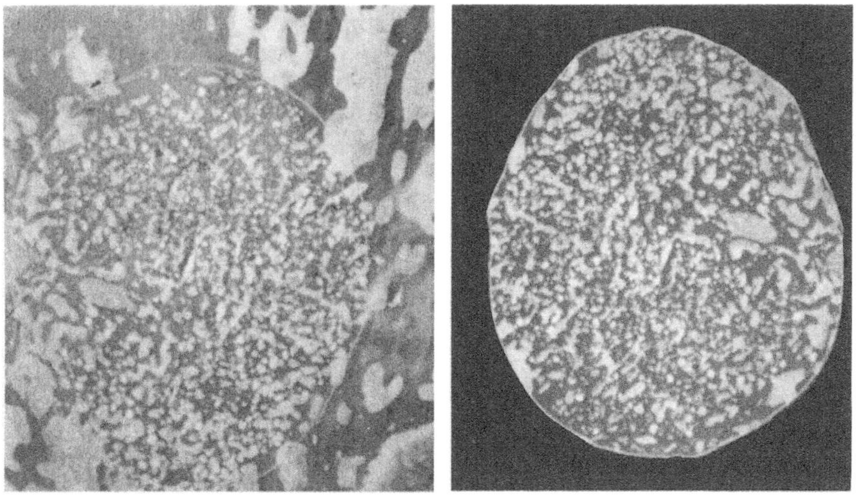

Fig. 5.10. Image analysis with IBAS (Kontron). The histological section appears on the monitor; the measuring sector is selected, and the surrounding area is suppressed

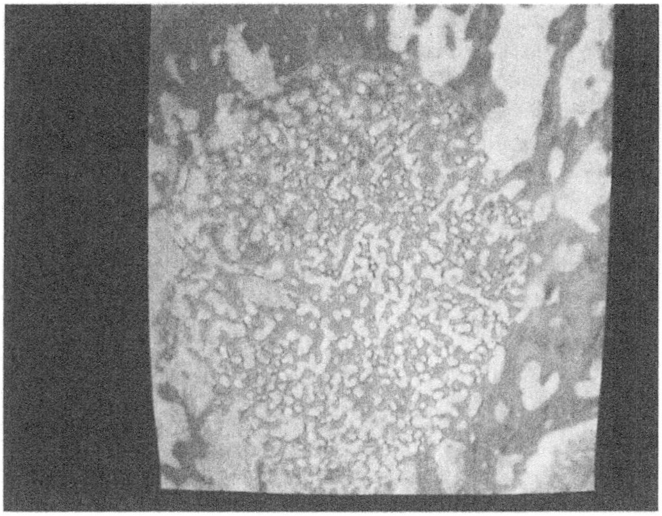

Fig. 5.11. The trabeculae to be determined are selected from the grey-shade scale, and the selection is checked again on the monitor

One disadvantage of this measuring technique, which needs to be mentioned, is that fully automatic histomorphometry is not capable of differentiating between newly grown and transplanted bone tissue. This is not, however, a problem when *implanting non-osseous* bone *components,* since in these tests *any bone* which is present *in the defect cavity* must necessarily be *regenerated* bone.

In the transplantation tests with autogenic spongiosa, we measured the transplanted spongiosa together with the regenerated bone. This is considered acceptable, because it can be expected that the transplanted autogenic spongiosa will be largely incorporated in the course of time. In preliminary pilot experiments, we attempted to distinguish between transplanted and newly grown bone by means of intravital polychrome fluorescence staining. These attempts, however, were not successful since the rapid growth of fibrous bone tissue led to diffuse staining, and the transplanted bone was also a partly stained, so that reliable differentiation between transplanted and newly grown bone was not possible. Standard polychrome sequential staining, on the other hand, yields good visibility of lamellar bone tissue, as demonstrated in the tests with cortical cross-sections.

5.4 Description of the Test Series

A total of 192 "cavity tests" on 96 rabbits were performed. In each rabbit, *both femoral condyles were compared.* The individual rabbits were given consecutive numbers from 1–96; rabbits 49–54 and 61–66 were used for pilot experiments, and were therefore excluded. This study thus consists of *168 tests* on a total of *84 rabbits.* For the sake of correct record-keeping, the consecutive numbers originally assigned to the animals were retained, and test animals 49–54 and 61–66 were ignored in this report.

Test animals 1–12 received an implant of small ceramised apatite granules (Apagran) in loose form without a carrier into the left femoral condyle, and the substance defect in the right femoral condyle was filled with an industrially manufactured collagen/powdered apatite mixed preparation in a weight ratio of 1:2 (Collapat B).

Test animals 13–24 received an implant into the left femoral condyle consisting of protein-free, pyrolysed and sintered natural calcium-phosphate ceramic material (Pyrost) and the usual commercial type of Kiel bone spongiosa splinters into the right condyle.

In test animals 25–36, the defect in the right femoral condyle was left empty, and the defect in the left femoral condyle was filled with allogenic "bone matrix".

In test animals 37–42, the defect in the right femoral condyle was left empty, and the left femoral condyle filled with an industrially manufactured collagen/apatite mixture (Collapat D) containing small granules of ceramised apatite (Apagran) instead of powdered apatite. The collagen-web carrier was, however, the same as used in tests 1–12.

Test animals 43–48 and 55–60 received particulate gelatin in both the left and the right femoral condyles; material from Merck was used in the left condyle, and material from Riedel, in the right condyle.

Test animals 67–80 received unilateral implantations of the further-improved collagen/apatite mixture (Collapat E), which again contained small ceramised apatite granules, but in which the collagen web exhibited secondary structural stabilisation due to cross-linking (cf. Sect. 4.4). The cavities on the other side were left empty and used as controls. The decision as to which side to fill and which side to leave empty in each animal was arrived at by tossing a coin.

In rabbits 81 and 82, the defect on the left-hand side was filled with Collapat E, and the defect on the right-hand side was filled with gelatin from Merck.

In animals 83 and 84, Ceros-80 Granulate, a porous hydroxyapatite ceramic material (Synthes) was implanted on the left side; the right cavity was left empty in rabbit 83, and was filled with Collapat E in rabbit 84.

In rabbits 85–96, the substance defect in the left femoral condyle was filled with autogenous spongiosa, and the right side was filled with collagen/apatite mixture (Collapat E).

All animal experiments were performed by the author himself.

Tables 5.2–5.9 give a detailed survey of the test series with test numbers and weights of the rabbits, implant material, post-operative observation period and complications.

5.4.1 Preparation of Implants

The collagen web/apatite preparations were obtained radiationsterilised and sealad from Osteo, ad could therefore be operatively implanted without further preparation. This applies to the collagen web with powdered apatite (Collapat B), the collagen web with

Table 5.2. Implantation of Collapat B and Apagran

Test	Weight (kg)	Implant material	Time	Complications
1R	4.0	Collapat B	6 weeks	—
1L		Apagran		—
2R	4.2	Collapat B	6 weeks	—
2L		Apagran		—
3R	3.2	Collapat B	4 weeks	Knee synovitis
3L		Apagran		—
4R	4.4	Collapat B	8 weeks	—
4L		Apagran		—
5R	3.5	Collapat B	4 weeks	—
5L		Apagran		—
6R	3.6	Collapat B	8 weeks	—
6L		Apagran		—
7R	3.6	Collapat B	8 months	Perforation
7L		Apagran		—
8R	4.0	Collapat B	2 weeks	Infection
8L		Apagran		—
9R	5.2	Collapat B	2 weeks	—
9L		Apagran		—
10R	4.0	Collapat B	4 weeks	Intra-operative bleeding
10L		Apagran		—
11R	4.0	Collapat B	11 days	—
11L		Apagran		Infection
12R	4.4	Collapat B	6 days	Death
12L		Apagran		—

R, right; L, left

Table 5.3. Implantation of Kiel bone splinters and Pyrost

Test	Weight (kg)	Implant material	Time	Complications
13R	3.0	Kiel bone	8 weeks	—
13L		Pyrost		—
14R	2.8	Kiel bone	8 weeks	—
14L		Pyrost		—
15R	4.0	Kiel bone	8 months	—
15L		Pyrost		—
16R	3.6	Kiel bone	3 months	—
16L		Pyrost		—
17R	3.0	Kiel bone	4 weeks	—
17L		Pyrost		—
18R	3.2	Kiel bone	4 weeks	—
18L		Pyrost		—
19R	4.0	Kiel bone	3 months	—
19L		Pyrost		—
20R	3.2	Kiel bone	2 weeks	—
20L		Pyrost		—
21R	2.9	Kiel bone	6 weeks	—
21L		Pyrost		—
22R	3.8	Kiel bone	6 weeks	—
22L		Pyrost		—
23R	3.6	Kiel bone	4 weeks	Death
23L		Pyrost		—
24R	3.5	Kiel bone	2 weeks	—
24L		Pyrost		—

R, right; L, left

small ceramised apatite granules of 100–150 μm diameter (Collapat D) and the structure-stabilised, cross-linked collagen web with small ceramised apatite granules of 50–150 μm diameter (Collapat E). In the case of Collapat B, the weight ratio of apatite to collagen was 2:1; with Collapat D and Collapat E it was 5:1.

During the operation, the autogenic spongiosa was removed from the opposite femoral condyle by means of a cylindrical cutter. The cylindrical cutter has an external diameter of 6 mm and an internal diameter of slightly more than 4 mm, so that the excised cylinders of autogenous spongiosa had an external diameter of just over 4 mm. The spongiosa cylinders could readily be pushed out of the cutter with a piston like rod.

The Kiel bone splinters were obtained sterilised and enclosed in a double-welded pack from Braun-Melsungen.

The bone matrix, Ceros 80, gelatin from Merck and Riedel, the non-embedded apatite granules of 150–250 μm (Apagran) and the deproteinated, pyrolised and sintered natural calcium-phosphate ceramic material (Pyrost) were transferred into plastic film, which was double welded, and gas sterilised with ethylene oxide (Gewalt and Fischer 1959; Fischer 1971). After gas sterilisation, all implantation materials were thoroughly aired in

Table 5.4. Implantation of allogenic "bone matrix" (BMP) and empty femoral condyle controls

Test	Weight (kg)	Implant material	Time	Complications
25R	3.4	Empty	6 weeks	—
25L		Matrix		—
26R	3.6	Empty	6 weeks	—
26L		Matrix		—
27R	4.0	Empty	8 weeks	—
27L		Matrix		—
28R	3.6	Empty	8 weeks	—
28L		Matrix		—
29R	3.8	Empty	3 months	—
29L		Matrix		—
30R	3.5	Empty	3 months	—
30L		Matrix		—
31R	4.0	Empty	2 weeks	—
31L		Matrix		—
32R	4.2	Empty	2 weeks	—
32L		Matrix		—
33R	4.2	Empty	4 weeks	—
33L		Matrix		—
34R	4.4	Empty	4 weeks	—
34L		Matrix		—
35R	2.8	Empty	8 months	—
35L		Matrix		—
36R	3.8	Empty	2 days	Paraplegia
36L		Matrix		Killed

R, right; L, left

the steriliser and then stored for 14 days under ambient conditions, so that one may assume that no residual ethylene oxide, which could possibly have an adverse effect on bone regeneration, remained in the implant materials.

Preparation of decalcified, devitalised and degreased *bone matrix* as an allogenic implant was performed by the author according to the procedure of Thielemann (personal communication), as follows: the femoral diaphyses of healthy rabbits were first cleaned, as thoroughly as possible, of all soft tissues. Following this, the femoral diaphyses were degreased for 24 h in methanol plus chloroform (1:1). The cortical bone structures were then broken up in a mortar, with bone scissors, to a size of less than 2000 μm. The cortical splinters obtained in this manner were degreased again in methanol and chloroform (1:1), the methanol-chloroform solution being changed several times during the process. Before each solvent change – and this applies also to the following steps – the remaining bone material was separated from the solution by filtering with a paper filter.

The splinters were then stirred for 24 h in 0.6 *N* HCl solution at 4 °C, the HCl solution being changed three times. Then followed 12 h treatment with 2 *M* $CaCl_2$, which was

Table 5.5. Implantation of Collapat D and empty femoral condyle controls respectively

Test	Weight (kg)	Implant material	Time	Complications
37R	3.3	Empty	6 weeks	—
37L		Collapat D		—
38R	3.0	Empty	2 weeks	—
38L		Collapat D		—
39R	4.1	Empty	6.5 weeks	—
39L		Collapat D		—
40R	3.2	Empty	4 weeks	—
40L		Collapat D		—
41R	3.0	Empty	2 weeks	—
41L		Collapat D		Infection
42R	3.2	Empty	4 weeks	—
42L		Collapat D		—

R, right; L, left

Table 5.6. Implantation of gelatin

Test	Weight (kg)	Implant material	Time	Complications
43R	3.2	Gelatin R	8 weeks	—
43L		Gelatin M		—
44R	3.6	Gelatin R	2 weeks	—
44L		Gelatin M		—
45R	3.0	Gelatin R	8 weeks	—
45L		Gelatin M		—
46R	2.6	Gelatin R	8 months	—
46L		Gelatin M		—
47R	2.6	Gelatin R	2 weeks	—
47L		Gelatin M		—
48R	3.2	Gelatin R	8 months	—
48L		Gelatin M		—
55R	3.4	Gelatin R	4 weeks	—
55L		Gelatin M		—
56R	3.2	Gelatin R	4 weeks	—
56L		Gelatin M		—
57R	3.2	Gelatin R	12 weeks	—
57L		Gelatin M		—
58R	3.8	Gelatin R	12 weeks	—
58L		Gelatin M		—
59R	3.2	Gelatin R	6 weeks	—
59L		Gelatin M		—
60R	4.1	Gelatin R	6 weeks	Death
60L		Gelatin M		—

Gelatin R was obtained from Riedel; Gelatin M was obtained from Merck. R, right; L, left

Table 5.7. Implantation of Collapat E, control side left empty

Test	Weight (kg)	Implant material	Time	Complications
67R	2.5	Empty	4 weeks	—
67L		Collapat E		—
68R	2.6	Collapat E	4 weeks	—
68L		Empty		—
69R	2.6	Empty	2 weeks	—
69L		Collapat E		—
70R	2.8	Collapat E	8 weeks	—
70L		Empty		—
71R	2.6	Collapat E	2 weeks	Infection
71L		Empty		Infection
72R	3.0	Collapat E	8 weeks	—
72L		Empty		—
73R	2.8	Collapat E	12 weeks	—
73L		Empty		—
74R	3.2	Collapat E	5 weeks	—
74L		Empty		—
75R	2.8	Empty	5 weeks	—
75L		Collapat E		—
76R	2.6	Empty	12 weeks	—
76L		Collapat E		—
77R	2.8	Empty	7.5 months	Death
77L		Collapat E		—
78R	2.8	Collapat E	8 months	—
78L		Empty		—
79R	2.9	Empty	3 weeks	—
79L		Collapat E		—
80R	2.9	Empty	3 weeks	—
80L		Collapat E		—

R, right; L, left

adjusted to pH 6, with stirring at 4 °C. The supernatant was then treated in 0.1 *M* EDTA solution for 12 h at 4 °C, followed by stirring for a further 12 h at 4 °C in 8 *M* $LiCl_2$ solution.

The supernatant was then washed and cleaned several times with distilled water at 50 °C. The remaining material was then lyophilised, packed into glass flasks, sealed and sterilised with ethylene oxide, then aired as described above, and stored at room temperature until it was used.

5.4.2 Results

5.4.2.1 Empty Cavities

Of course, in assessing the effects of bone-replacement materials, the applicability of the experimental model to the question being investigated is of paramount importance.

Table 5.8. Implantation of autogenic spongiosa and Collapat E

Test	Weight (kg)	Implant material	Time	Complications
85R	3.1	Collapat E	4 weeks	Condylar fracture
85L		Autogenic spongiosa		—
86R	2.6	Collapat E	4 weeks	—
86L		Autogenic spongiosa		Condylar fracture
87R	2.8	Collapat E	4 weeks	—
87L		Autogenic spongiosa		—
88R	3.0	Collapat E	26 days	Death
88L		Autogenic spongiosa		—
89R	2.6	Collapat E	4 weeks	—
89L		Autogenic spongiosa		—
90R	3.4	Collapat E	4 weeks	—
90L		Autogenic spongiosa		—
91R	3.2	Collapat E	3 weeks	—
91L		Autogenic spongiosa		—
92R	4.2	Collapat E	3 weeks	—
92L		Autogenic spongiosa		—
93R	4.2	Collapat E	3 weeks	—
93L		Autogenic spongiosa		—
94R	3.0	Collapat E	3 weeks	—
94L		Autogenic spongiosa		—
95R	3.4	Collapat E	3 weeks	—
95L		Autogenic spongiosa		—
96R	4.5	Collapat E	3 weeks	—
96L		Autogenic spongiosa		—

R, right; L, left

Since the rabbit is reported to have a very high bone-regeneration capacity, we devoted particular attention to spontaneous bone regeneration in our animal model and carried out a total of 32 control experiments. Of these, 12 were run in direct comparison to bone matrix, 6 to Collapat D and 14 to Collapat E, between 2 weeks and 8 months after implantation.

From literature reports about the very good callous-forming capacity of the rabbit, one would have been led to expect that empty bone defects would, sooner or later, be filled up spontaneously with bone. Surprisingly, this was *not* the case, as had already been pointed out by Nizard (1981).

This is the first noteworthy result of our own experimental work to be confirmed in a quantitatively exact manner. The formation of new bone in the empty cavities remained restricted to the edge of the defect, and the largest part at the centre of the defect remained free of bone during the entire course of the test, i.e. up to 8 months, and was filled with bone marrow rich in fat cells. At the edge of the defect – and only there – vigorous growth of new bone, which led to remarkable thickening and reinforcement of the area at the edge of the defect, was observed. The weakening of the bone segment by

Table 5.9. Implantation of Collapat E, Gelatin M or Ceros 80 and empty condyles

Test	Weight (kg)	Implant material	Time (weeks)	Complications
81R	2.9	Gelatin M	1	—
81L		Collapat E		—
82R	2.6	Gelatin M	1	—
82L		Collapat E		—
83R	3.1	Empty	3	—
83L		Ceros 80		—
84R	2.6	Collapat E	4	—
84L		Ceros 80		—

Gelatin M was obtained from Merck. R, right; L, left

Tabele 5.10. Average spontaneous bone regeneration measured in the empty cavities

Test number	Test period (weeks)	Regenerated bone measured per unit area (%)
31R	2	8.2
32R	2	7.1
41R	2	5.6
38R	2	6.1
69R	2	9.4
71L	2	8.6
33R	4	1.9
34R	4	3.4
42R	4	1.7
67R	4	12.6
68L	4	9.4
25R	6	2.4
26R	6	0.3
37R	6	10.9
39R	6	0.6
74L	6	10.2
75R	6	3.0
27R	8	31.9
28R	8	9.3
70L	8	3.4
72L	8	1.6
73L	12	10.1
76R	12	8.6
29R	12	10.3
78L	32	16.7

R, right condyle; L, left condyle

the introduction of the defect cavity was obviously at least partially compensated by this *thickening at the edge.* Clearly, the well-known callous-forming capacity of the rabbit does not become effective in this test model. Since the bone defect chosen in the rabbit, with a size of 6 mm, cannot be filled spontaneously with regenerated bone, **this test model**

may be regarded as suitable for the scope of this work, and the widespread prejudice against the use of rabbits in bone-regeneration studies can be considered unjustified in the case of the particular test model which we used.

Since the bone-regeneration studies carried out by Schweiberer (1970) in the dog demonstrate conclusively that the dog is capable of closing even a 10 mm defect with regenerated bone within about 3 weeks, it can even be concluded that **drilled 6 mm cavities in the rabbit allow a better assessment of bone regeneration under the influence of different implantation materials than 10 mm drilled cavities in the dog.** The statements are given additional credibility by the results of *quantitative determinations of spontaneous bone regeneration in empty cavities.* The values for the relative surface area of regenerated bone in the defect cavity, in relation to the total surface being evaluated, can be found in Table 5.10. For various reasons (artefacts, unsatisfactory sections, eccentric defect cavities), not all experiments could be quantitatively evaluated.

For rabbits 67–78, ten sections per specimen were made from different section planes at intervals of 50 μm. All ten sections were measured. From the ten values obtained, the average was calculated and listed in Table 5.10. For the remaining rabbits, three different sections per specimen were made and evaluated accordingly. The average values are also listed in Table 5.10.

The *amount* of bone grown in the individual rabbits *varied* impressively, as one would expect to find in a biological experiment. This again underlines the importance of quantitative evaluation. The regenerated bone in the empty cavities varied between a minimum of 0.3% and a maximum of 31.9%, with an average of 8.5%. Of the 25 empty cavities evaluated, 18 showed new bone formation below 10%. Four showed bone growth between 10% and 15%, and only three exhibited bone growth of more than 15% (Fig. 5.12).

When the results obtained are evaluated as a function of time, it becomes apparent that between 2 weeks and 8 months, the time elapsed after implantation had practically

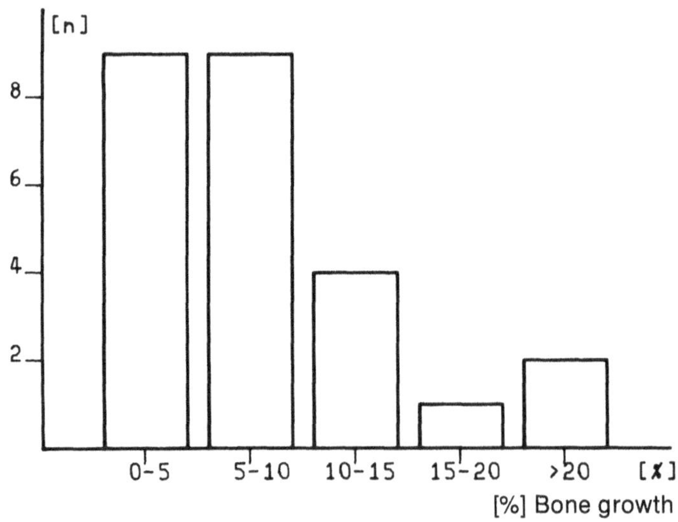

Fig. 5.12. Bone regeneration in empty cavities ($n = 25$). Most cavities show only very slight peripheral bone regeneration

no influence on the amount of regenerated bone present. In other words, *progressive bony reconstruction of the defect cavity with the course of time was not detected.*

In *long term experiments,* the bone defect was *still clearly visible after 8 months.* Control experiments with a duration of less than 2 weeks were not considered necessary, since other experiments had already shown that bone regeneration only starts in the second week, although once it starts it proceeds very rapidly and massively. The control experiments served as a basis for the assessment of bone regeneration under the influence of different implantation materials. Reference will be made to these control experiments in the following chapters (Figs. 5.13–5.15).

5.4.2.2 Autogenic Spongiosa

In the present investigation, 11 transplantations of autogenic spongiosa were performed. Apart from the control experiments, we considered that it was important to compare the effects of bone-replacement materials with those of autogenic spongiosa. This permits a *direct comparison* of the *best bone-transplant* material with the *most suitable bone-replacement* material (Fig. 5.16).

Earlier tests had shown that bone regeneration starts in week 2, reaches a maximum in week 3 and ends in week 4. Thereafter essentially only bone-remodelling processes can be observed. We therefore limited the test duration to 3–4 weeks in the implantation experiments with autogenic spongiosa, but evaluated twelve rabbits. In one of the 3-week experiments, however, it was impossible to cut out a suitable autogenic spongiosa cylinder with the cylindrical cutter. In this case, we performed an *allogenic* spongiosa transplant.

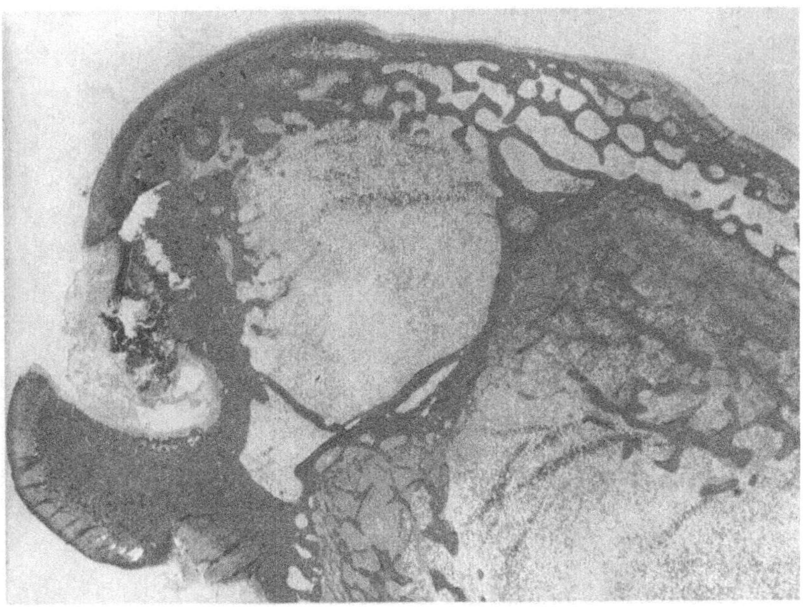

Fig. 5.13. Empty cavity after 6 weeks (test 74). Bony reinforcement of the peripheral structures has occurred; the defect persists

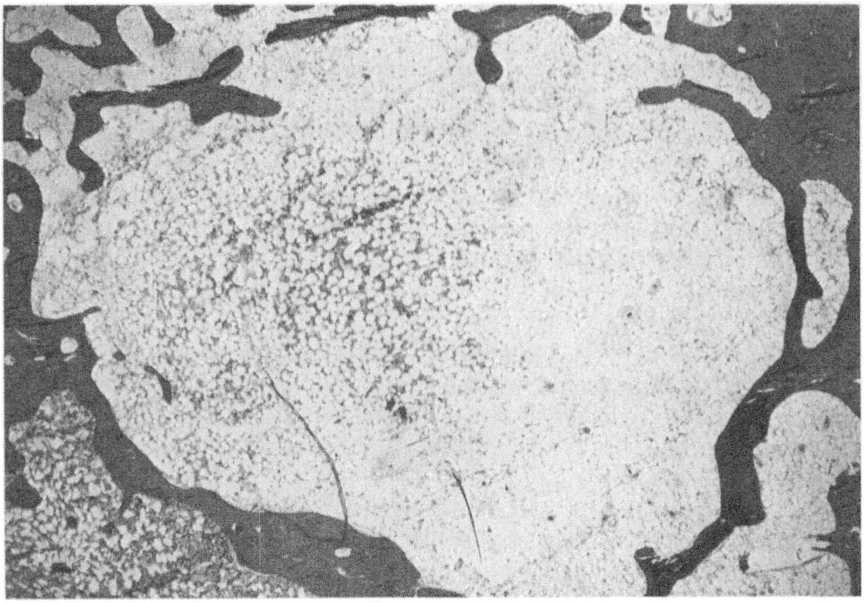

Fig. 5.14. The empty bone defect persists for a long time. The rabbit bone used in our test model is obviously not capable of spontaneous regeneration. (Test 29 right, empty cavity, 12 weeks) Masson-Goldner (MG), × 15

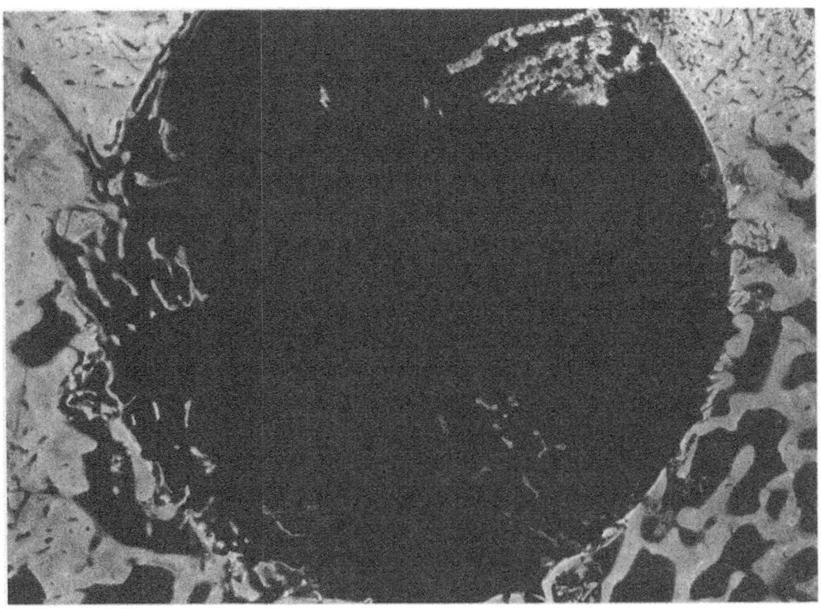

Fig. 5.15. Slight peripheral bone regeneration. (Test 41 right, empty cavity, 2 weeks, microradiograph) × 15

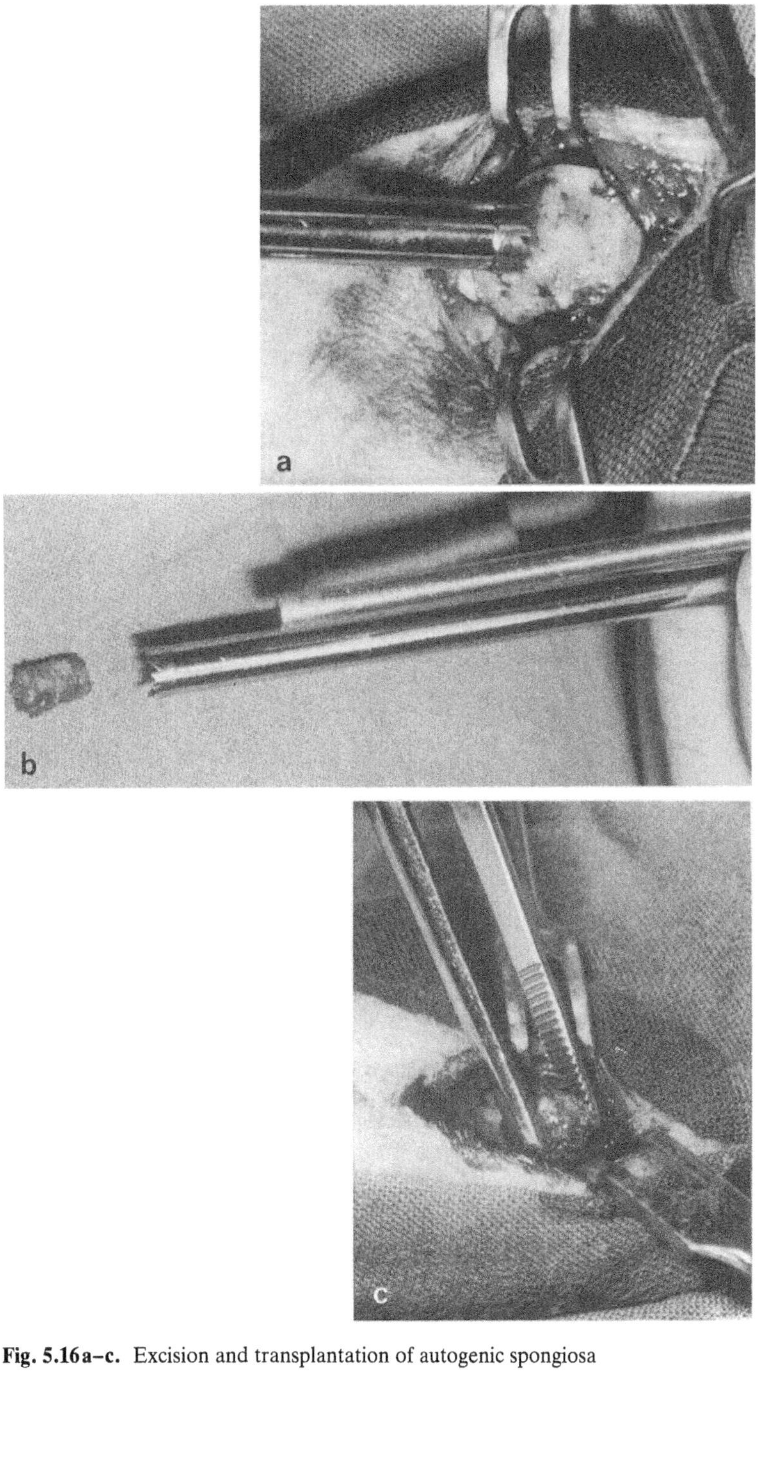

Fig. 5.16a–c. Excision and transplantation of autogenic spongiosa

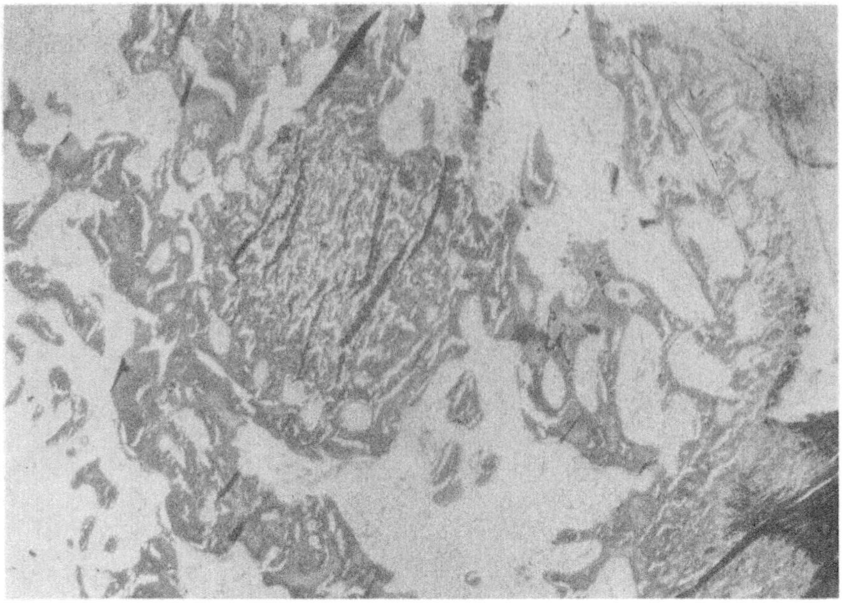

Fig. 5.17. Dense bony growth filling up the defect containing compact spongy transplantate (Test 89 left, 4 weeks) MG, × 15

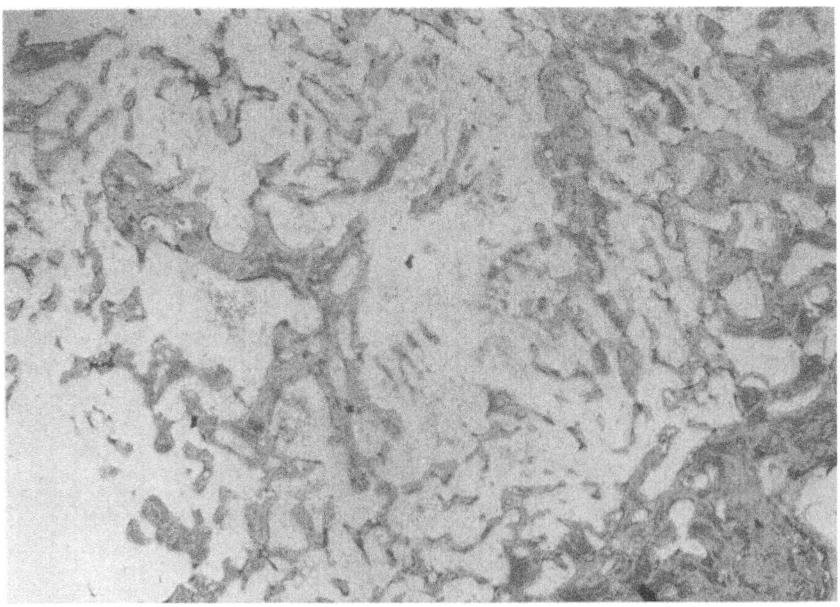

Fig. 5.18. Wide-meshed, comparatively sparse bony reconstruction after autogenous spongiosa transplantation (Test 91 left, 3 weeks) MG, × 15

It was not with in the scope of this project to study (yet again) bone regeneration under the influence of autogenic spongiosa, since sufficient investigations of this subject already exist. The evaluation of autogenic spongiosa was therefore limited to quantitative and qualitative assessment after 3 and 4 weeks (Figs. 5.17 and 5.18). We considered this to be a better procedure, as it enabled us to evaluate the maximal number of test animals during the most interesting time period (Figs. 5.19 and 5.20).

The results of these tests after 3 weeks showed that *transplanted autogenous spongiosa survives and is integrated*. Many blood vessels could be seen in the vicinity of the transplanted spongy trabeculae. *Massive numbers of osteoblasts* with small osteoid seams were found all over the spongy trabeculae in the defect cavity. On the surface of the transplanted spongy trabeculae, bone growth by apposition was taking place. Occasionally new bone tissue was detected in the marrow independently of the transplanted spongiosa; otherwise, however, the spaces between the spongy trabeculae were filled with blood vessels and marrow tissue; sometimes a fibrous scar was also present. In contrast to the quiescence of the marrow tissue in the intact surroundings, the abundance of cells and blood vessels in the spaces between the spongy trabeculae in the bone defect was typical of intensive repair processes (Figs. 5.19–5.21). Necrotic spongy trabeculae and osteoblasts were detected only very occasionally.

In contrast to this, formation of new bone was observed only at the edge of the defect in the rabbit which had received an *allogenic spongiosa transplantation*. Abacterial inflammatory infiltrations and necrotic bone trabeculae, which were torn out during the cutting process, were also found. This was obviously an immunological response.

In autogenic spongiosa transplantation, the findings after 4 weeks were much the same as after 3 weeks, but in some cases there were considerably fewer osteoblasts on the

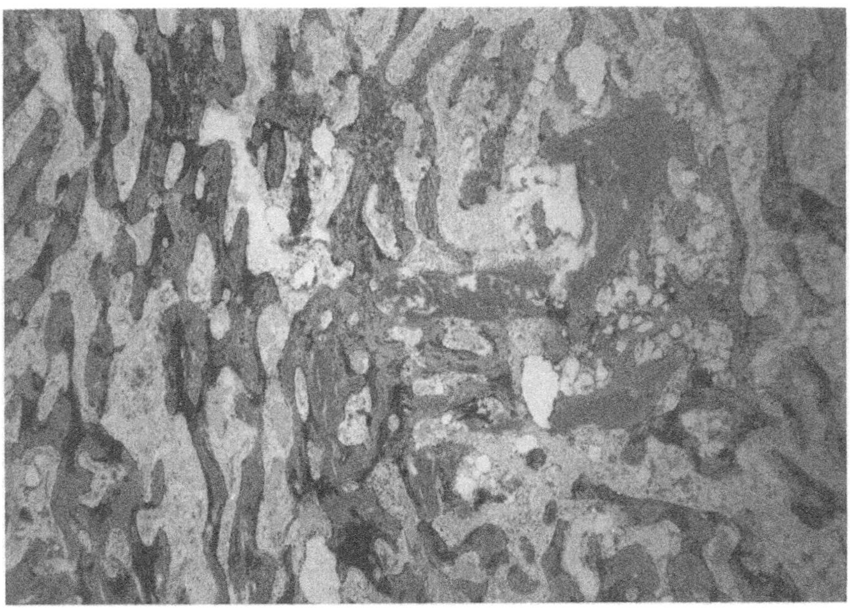

Fig. 5.19. Autogenic spongiosa transplantation with vigorous bone regeneration (Test 92 left, 3 weeks) MG, × 25

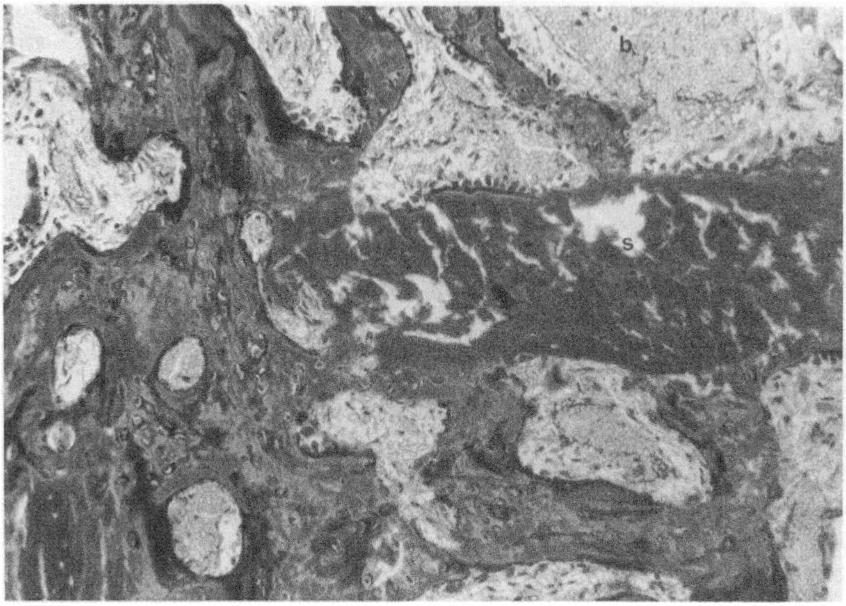

Fig. 5.20. Magnification of a sector with abundant blood vessels (b) and new bone tissue (k) on the surface of the transplanted spongiosa (s). × 100

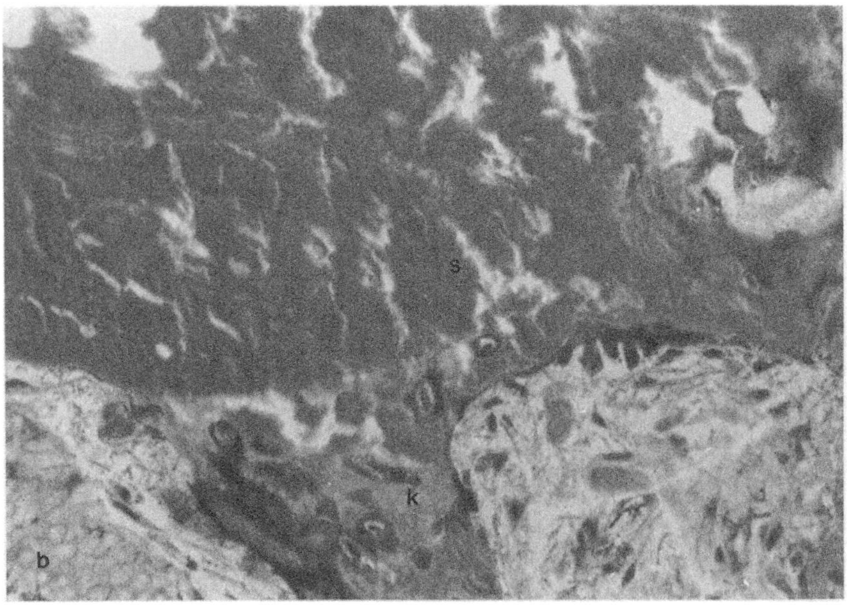

Fig. 5.21. Enlargement of a sector from Fig. 5.20, showing partly necrotic osteocytes in the transplanted spongiosa (s) and partial residual staining of the nucleus. On the surface are newly formed bony trabeculae (k). Adjacent blood vessels are seen (b). × 300

surfaces of the spongy trabeculae. In these cases, the regeneration process had obviously ended (Figs. 5.22–5.23).

As has been explained already in Sect 5.3.8, quantitative analysis using the automated image-analysis system is not capable of differentiating between regenerated and transplanted bone, so that a *quantitative determination registers both transplanted material and regenerated bone in the same manner.* This seems justified in the case of autogenic transplants, because the transplanted material survives, is largely incorporated, and is thus equivalent to new bone tissue.

As explained above, our attempt to achieve accurate colourimetric differentiation between regenerated and transplanted bone by means of polychromic fluorescence staining was not successful. The difficulty – as previously shown by Schenk and Willenegger (1977) – is that rapid and expansive fibrous-bone formation leads to diffuse, broad staining with fluorochromes, which makes calculation of the rate of bone apposition on the fibrous bone impossible.

Two tests had to be excluded from quantitative evaluation, due to fracture of the condyle. In a further test it was not possible to extract a suitable spongiosa cylinder with the cylindrical cutter, and for this reason an allogenic spongiosa transplant was performed in this instance. Naturally, this test also had to be excluded from the quantitative evaluation.

A total of nine tests could be quantitatively evaluated. Three different bone sections per test were evaluated, and these values were used to calculate the average. The calculated average proportional areas of bone surface in the nine defect cavities with autogenic spongiosa transplants evaluated showed a minimum of 23.3%, a maximum of 52.3% and an average of 32.4% (Table 5.11).

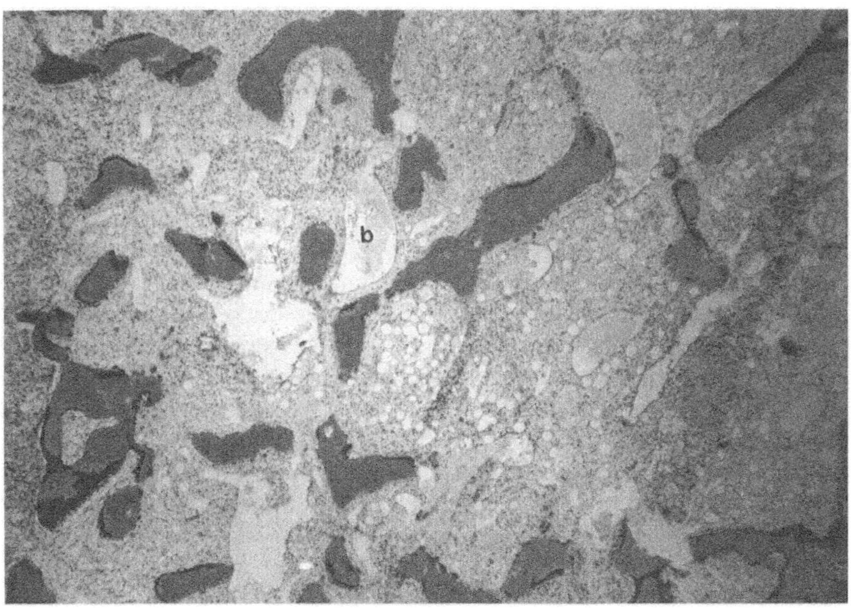

Fig. 5.22. Numerous blood vessels (*b*) around the transplanted spongiosa. Bone apposition has occurred on the surface of the spongiosa, but there has been little formation of new bone in the spaces. (Test 95 left, 3 weeks) MG, × 40

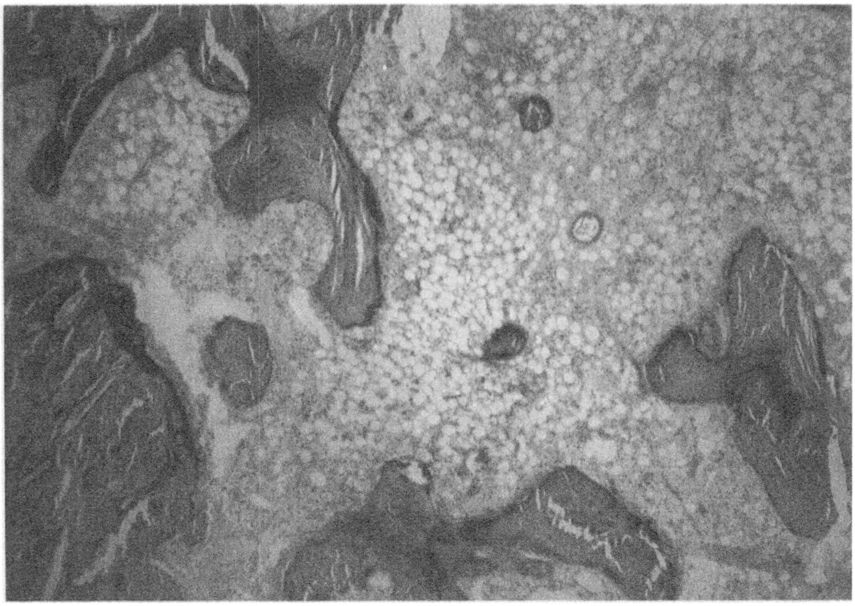

Fig. 5.23. Transplanted spongiosa with bone apposition. (Test 94 left, 3 weeks) MG, × 60

As expected, the relative amount of bone present was considerably higher after spongiosa transplantation than with defect cavities which were left empty. On average, about four times more bone was found after spongiosa transplantation than with empty cavities. These values served as a positive control in the assessment of bone-replacement materials.

5.4.2.3 Bone Matrix

In this group, a total of 12 implants were performed. The matrix, prepared and implanted according to Thielemann (personal communication), had a bright red colour in the slides with Masson-Goldner (MG) staining and a pale blue colour when stained according to Giemsa (Figs. 5.23 and 5.24). Figure 5.25 summarises the results obtained.

After *2 weeks,* new mineralised bone trabeculae could already be detected on the surface of the bone matrix. Some of these were laid down directly on the matrix, without formation of a separating interface layer, but sometimes they were separated from the matrix by a broad layer of connective tissue. Phagocytes were seen in many places, as well as many new blood vessels in the spaces and a fibrous scar. While one of the 2-week sections already showed narrow bone seams in many places on the matrix surface, in the second 2-week experiment very few new bony trabeculae were detected in the defect cavity (Figs. 5.26 and 5.27).

In one of the 4-week tests, almost no bone was found in the defect cavity, which contained mostly connective tissue and inflammatory infiltrate (Fig. 5.28). The second 4-week section showed occasional small areas of fibrous bone distributed throughout the entire defect cavity, partly on the surface of the matrix but partly separate from it. The largest section of the defect, however, showed no evidence of new bone formation.

Table 5.11. Surface-area measurement of new bone formation and of the transplanted spongiosa 3 and 4 weeks after filling with autogenic spongiosa

Test number	Test duration (weeks)	Bone formation measured per unit surface area (%)
91L	3	38.8
92L	3	37.8
93L	3	27.8
94L	3	26.9
95L	3	23.3
87L	4	32.3
88L	4	32.7
89L	4	52.3
90L	4	27.9

L, left

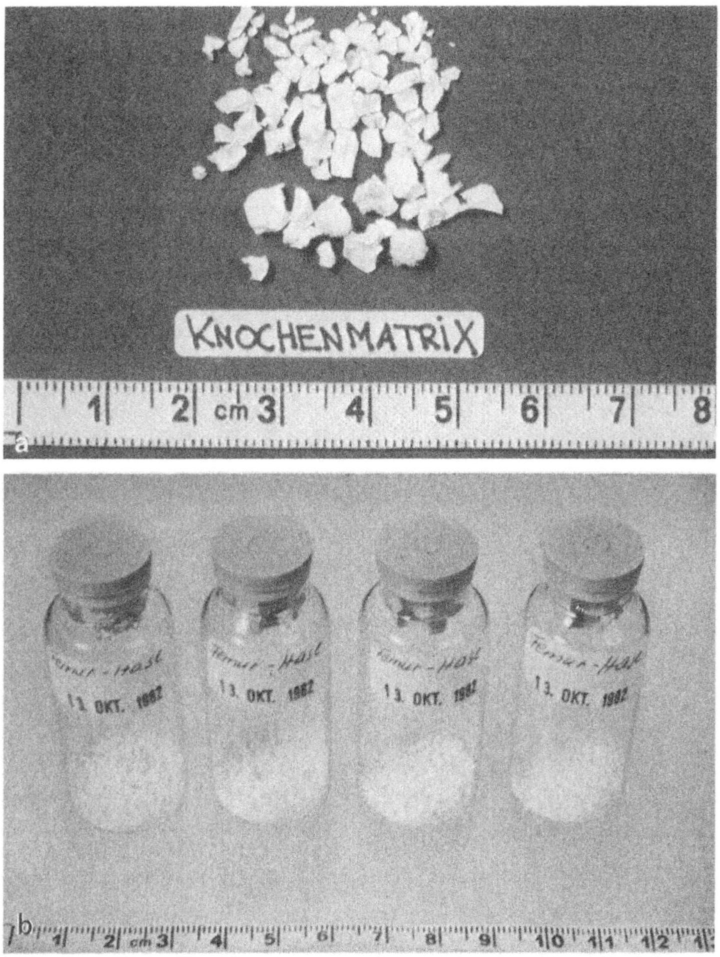

Fig. 5.24. a Macroscopic view of the allogenic bone matrix made in this laboratory according to the method of Urist (1965) (see text for procedure). **b** After lyophilisation in glass ampoules

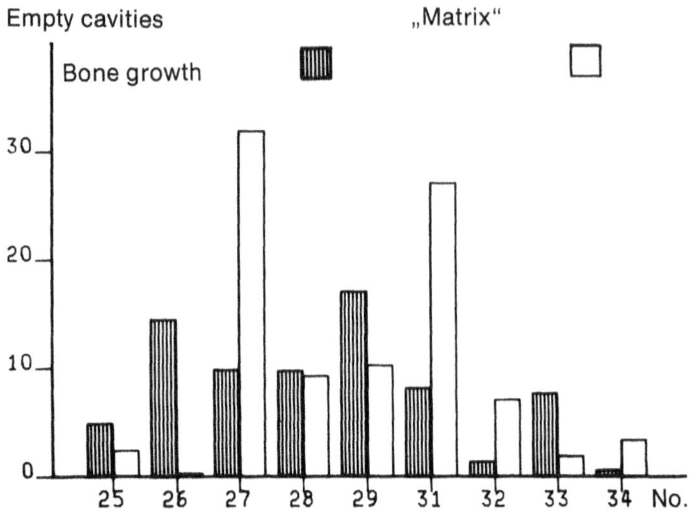

Fig. 5.25. Results of bone regeneration tests with "bone matrix" in comparison to empty cavities. The graph illustrates the fundamental differences, and underlines the need for quantitative evaluation. The difference in bone regeneration between matrix-filled and empty cavities was not statistically significant

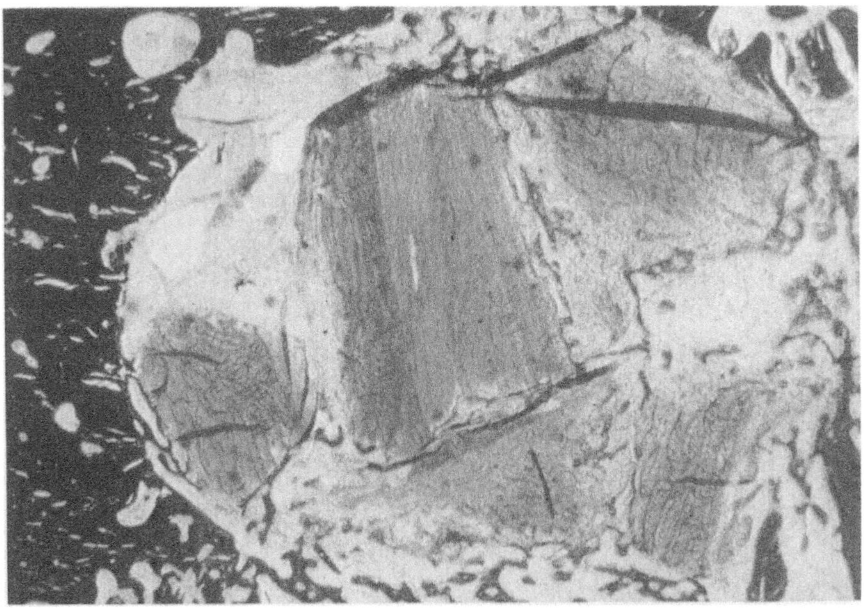

Fig. 5.26. Sporadic bone regeneration (dark) on the matrix surface (grey). (Test 31, 2 weeks) MG, × 15

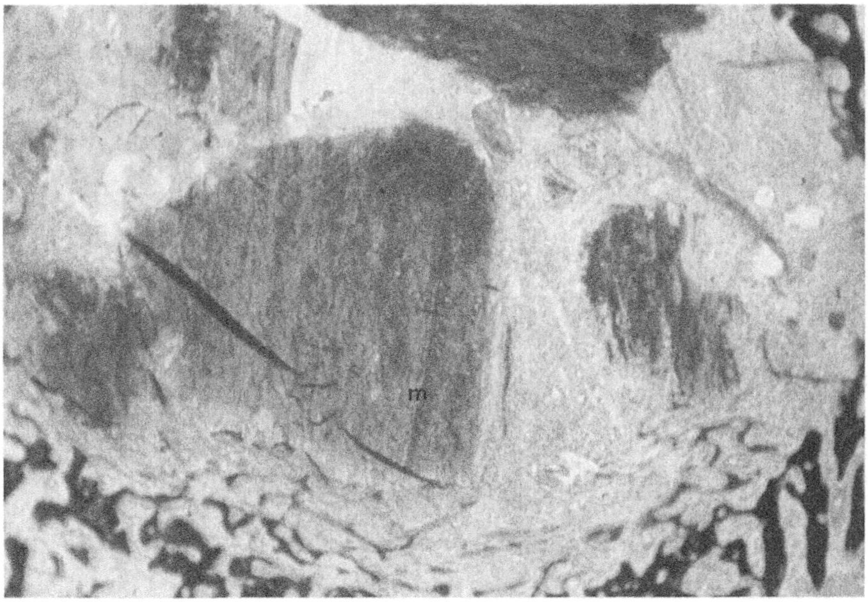

Fig. 5.27. The decalcified red matrix (*m*) shows only slight evidence of new bone formation on this surface. (Test 32 left, matrix, 2 weeks) MG, × 18

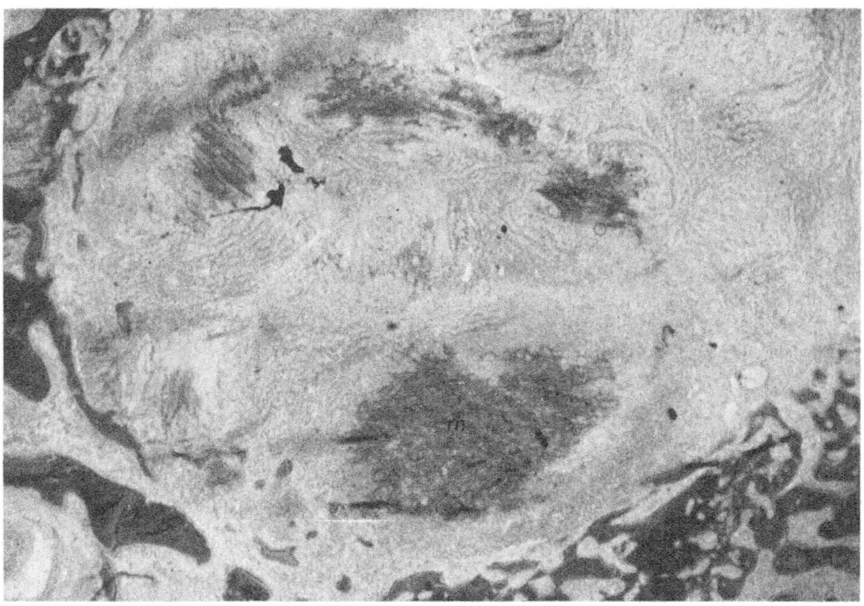

Fig. 5.28. The red matrix (*m*) is still clearly discernible. The amount of new bone growth remains disappointingly low. (Test 34 left, matrix, 4 weeks) MG, × 18

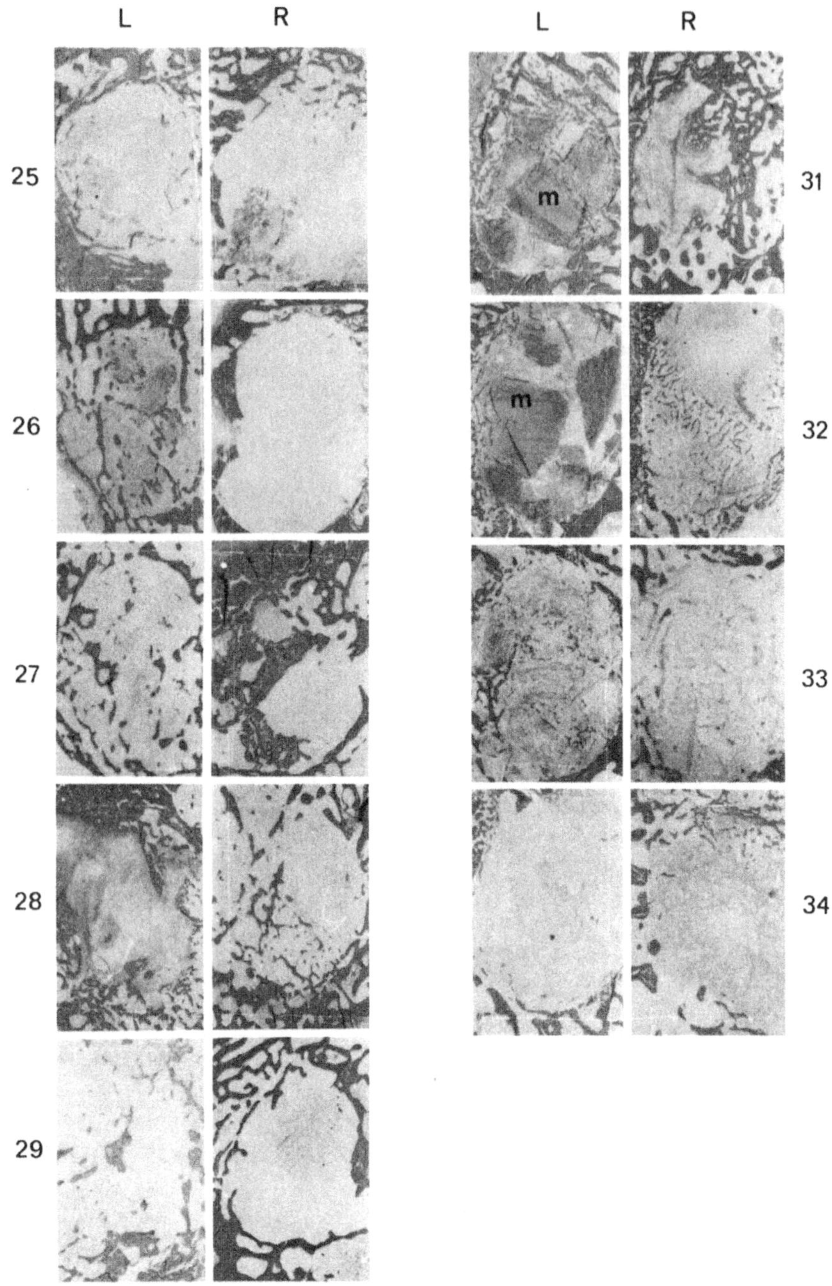

Fig. 5.29. Series of survey photographs, showing slight and incomplete bone regeneration with marked individual variation. The red matrix implants (*m*) have a grey colour in the black and white photographs, and should not be confused with bone tissue. *L,* bone matrix; *R* empty cavity. (2–12 weeks, *test number adjacent to the photograph*) MG, × 4

Even after *6 weeks,* the matrix implantate could still clearly be recognised as such, but was progressively being degraded. The histological appearance at this time was still predominantly that of cell-rich granulation tissue. The new bone trabeculae had not increased in quantity, but could still be detected sporadically, both in the centre of the defect and on the surface of the implant. Some of these small bone trabeculae still exhibited osteoblasts on their surface and showed evidence of further bone growth by apposition; we also found bone trabeculae without osteoblasts in the adjacent region where bone regeneration had obviously been completed. In the second 6-week test, however, peripheral new bone was only occasionally detectable.

After *8 weeks,* the matrix had been almost totally broken down, and the defect cavity was filled mainly by a *scar of connective tissue,* unlike the empty cavities, in which after the 4th week most of the defect was already filled with unremarkable bone-marrow tissue containing many fat cells.

After *12 weeks,* reconstruction had been completed; as well, the matrix implants had developed a normal bone marrow. Remnants of the matrix implants were no longer detectable. The boundaries of the bone defect were no longer clearly discernible, but the former defect area was *still characterised by a lack of bone.*

To summarise, we gained the impression that, in defect cavities filled with matrix implants, partial formation of new bone occurs on the matrix surface. Quantitative comparison with empty cavities on the opposite side showed, however, *that there was no statistically significant increase in bone growth* after matrix implantation. Nine tests could be evaluated quantitatively, and again three different bone sections per test were measured (Fig. 5.29).

The test results after matrix implantation varied from a minimum of 0.6% to a maximum of 17.1%, with an average of 8.2% (Table 5.12, Fig. 5.25).

No significant difference in bone regeneration **between empty cavities and matrix implantation** could be found in the Wilcoxon pair-difference test.

5.4.2.4 Kiel Bone Splinters

Twelve implants with Kiel bone splinters were carried out.

With Masson-Goldner staining, the Kiel bone splinters could be distinguished in preparations from the light green, newly formed bone trabeculae by their somewhat

Table 5.12. Influence of bone-matrix implantation on bone regeneration between 2 and 12 weeks

Test number	Test duration (weeks)	Bone formation measured per unit surface area (%)
31L	2	8.2
32L	2	1.4
33L	4	7.7
34L	4	0.6
25L	6	4.9
26L	6	14.5
27L	8	9.9
28L	8	9.8
29L	12	17.1

L, left

darker green colour. Obviously, the Kiel bone splinters are also *more fragile and brittle;* in contrast to the new bone trabeculae formed and the surrounding bone structures, they were sometimes peeled off the section during the cutting process. Furthermore, the osteocytic structures did not exhibit nuclear staining. With the Giemsa staining technique, the Kiel bone splinters acquired a pale-pink colour which was similar to the colour of the mature structures of the intact bone tissue. In contrast, the empty osteocytic cavities were separated from the pale-pink-stained mineralised bone tissues in the Kieler splinters by a narrow dark blue membrane, and residual osteocytic structures still appeared to be present. The Kiel bone splinters formed a loose lattice with wide gaps; the implant was made up of a wide-meshed spongy structure.

After *2 weeks,* many blood vessels had been formed in the gaps between the mesh of the Kiel spongy material, and there was also formation of new bone in the centre. New bone growth occurred *partly in contact with the Kiel bone splinters, but mostly separated from them.* Apart from this, significant amounts of connective-tissue scar were found to have grown into the cavity from the edge.

While, at 2 weeks, massive numbers of osteoblasts could be detected on the surfaces of the new bone trabeculae, and foci of initial formation of new bone in the marrow cavities were present, the bone-regeneration process had obviously been completed at *4 weeks.* Although new bone trabeculae were still present within the defect cavity, there were almost no osteoblasts on the surface. On the other hand, *granuloma-type cell agglomerations* could now be seen in several places in the vicinity of the Kiel bone spongiosa, and in some areas dense *lymphocytic infiltrations* were visible (Figs. 5.30–5.32). Also, the formation of connective tissue, which in one of the two sections filled the marrow cavities of the implant, had assumed a more prominent role, whereas the formation of new bone had become less important. It was obvious that the Kiel bone splinters had provoked a *violent defensive process,* which was leading to increasing resorption, both of the implanted material and the new bone trabeculae (Fig. 5.33).

After *8 months,* only *small residues* of the Kiel bone splinters could still be detected; most of the bone defect had been filled with fat-cell-rich marrow, which reverted to a normal appearance. In only one of the two sections made in week 12 was it still possible to see large amounts of Kiel bone within the defect, surrounded by a fibrous scar (Fig. 5.34).

The interpretation of these findings is that the (only partially) deproteinated Kiel bone splinters are not immunogen-free, despite reports to the contrary, and that they provoke an immunological defensive reaction which is almost undetectable at 2 weeks, but obviously reaches a maximum after 4 weeks. There seem to be individual differences; in some cases the Kieler material has already been resorbed after 6 weeks, and in some cases it can still be detected after 12 weeks. The **bone regeneration processes** which begin in week 2 **are stopped by this defensive reaction, so that eventually the histological picture is dominated by connective-tissue cicatrisation.** After resorption of the Kiel splinters, the connective tissue is replaced by marrow tissue, which at first contains many fat cells but then reverts back to an unremarkable appearance.

The difference in colour contrast between regenerated bone tissue and Kiel bone material can be detected visually with the microscope, but is so slight that the automatic image analyser cannot differentiate between implantate and regenerated bone. This is also true for *microradiography,* with which the difference in contrast between recently mineralised bone and Kiel bone is quite small. Quantitative evaluation of the test series was therefore not possible using the automatic image analyser. However, such quantita-

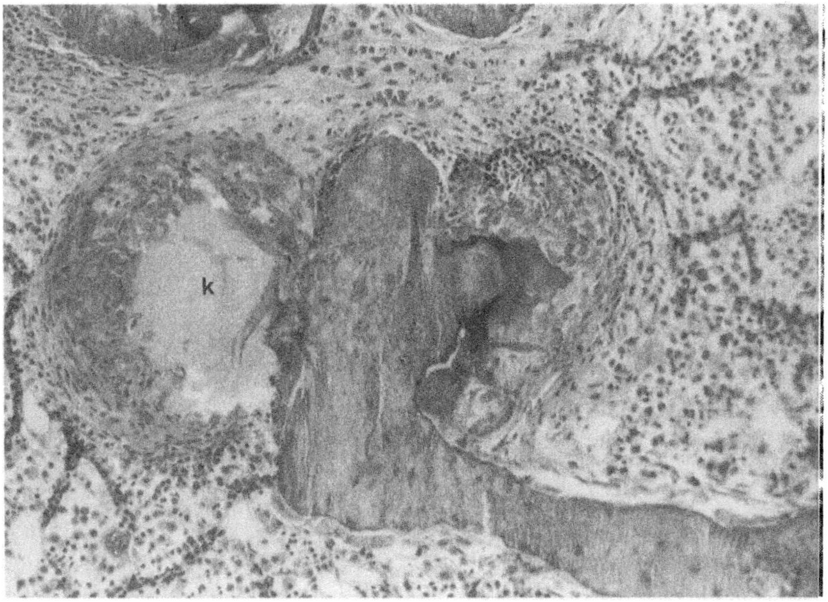

Fig. 5.30. Kiel bone splinter (*k*) surrounded by granuloma. Abacterial inflammatory infiltrates eventually degrade not only the implanted Kiel splinters, but also part of the regenerated bone. Test 17 right, 4 weeks) Giemsa, × 40

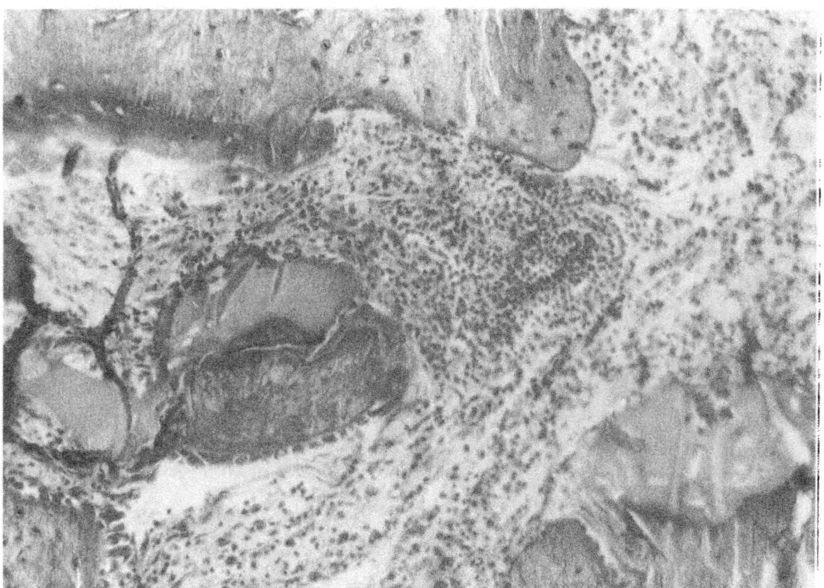

Fig. 5.31. Similar finding as in Fig. 5.30 in another sector. (Test 17 right, 4 weeks) Giemsa, × 40

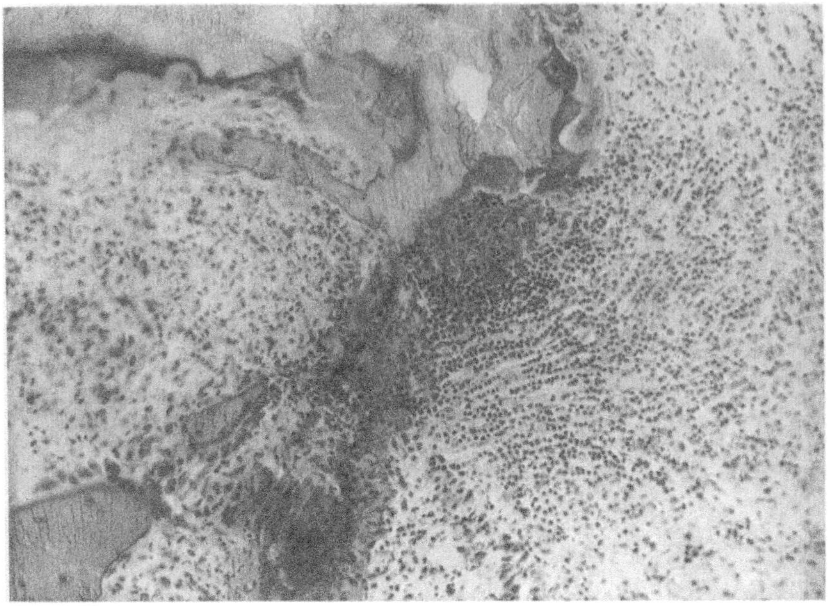

Fig. 5.32. Granulomatous inflammatory defence reaction after implantation of Kiel bone splinters, showing round-cell infiltration. (Test 18 right, 4 weeks) Giemsa, × 40

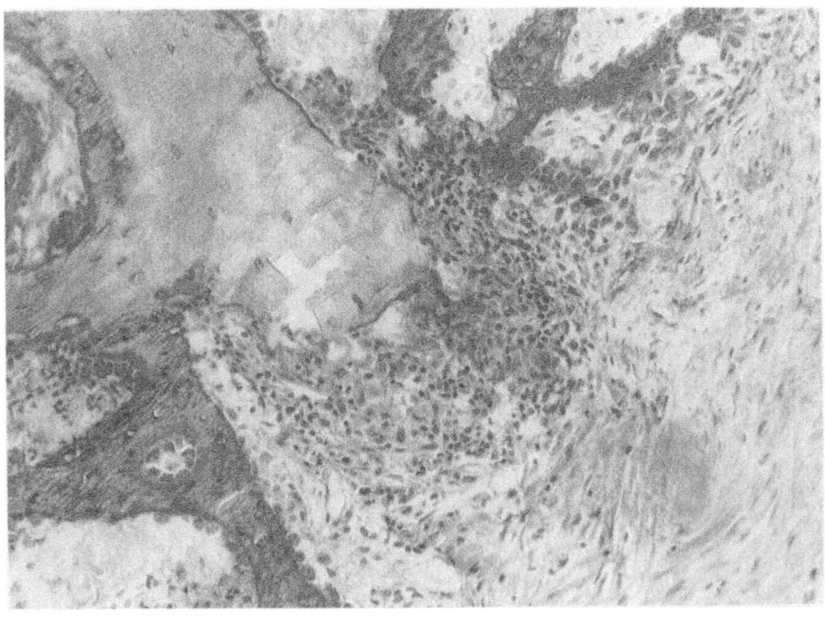

Fig. 5.33. Kiel bone splinters are attacked and eventually degraded by the immunological response to the tissue. The partly regenerated bone is also affected, as shown by the scar on the *right*. (Test 21 right, 6 weeks) Giemsa, × 40

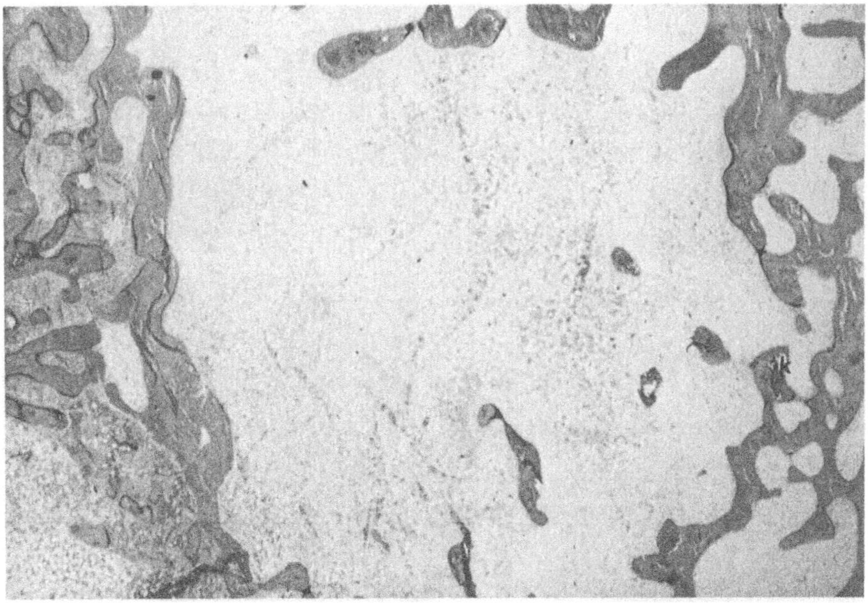

Fig. 5.34. Long-term result with Kiel bone splinters, after 8 months. The Kieler splinters have been completely resorbed except for minor residues (*k*), and the defect cavity contains practically no regenerated bone. (Test 15 right) MG, × 15

tive evaluation was not really necessary, since *qualitative* histological assessment of the slides had already shown the Kieler bone splinters to be unsuitable material.

5.4.2.5 Gelatin

In the left-right test we implanted and evaluated two different preparations of particulate gelatin in 12 animal experiments, so that a total of 24 gelatin implantations were carried out. The gelatin preparation obtained from Merck was implanted on the left, and that obtained from Riedel on the right side. We filled the defect cavities loosely, up to the edge, with gelatin particles. The particles from Merk (Art. No. 4078) were smaller than those from Riedel, and had an average size of 250 μm. The powdered gelatin from Riedel (Art. No. 18807, batch designation 3046) was coarser, and the particles had an average size of approximately 500 μm (Fig. 5.35).

Histology showed essentially no difference in the tissue reaction to the two gelatin preparations. After *2 weeks,* the entire defect cavity was filled with loose connective tissue which contained relatively few blood vessels. The cells present were predominantly fibrocytes. The *formation of new bone* in one of the two 2-week tests was limited to the outer edge of the defect; this was true both for the Merck and the Riedel implants. The other 2-week test showed moderate radial proliferation of new fibrous bone. The preparation seemed to be well tolerated by the tissue. It is remarkable that absolutely *no defensive reaction* foreign-body granuloma or round-cell infiltration was detected.

After *4 weeks,* the fibrous connective tissue receded; instead, unremarkable bone marrow with many fat cells appeared. However, the bone cavity remained *completely free of regenerated bone.* This applied for the entire test period of up to 8 months, with the

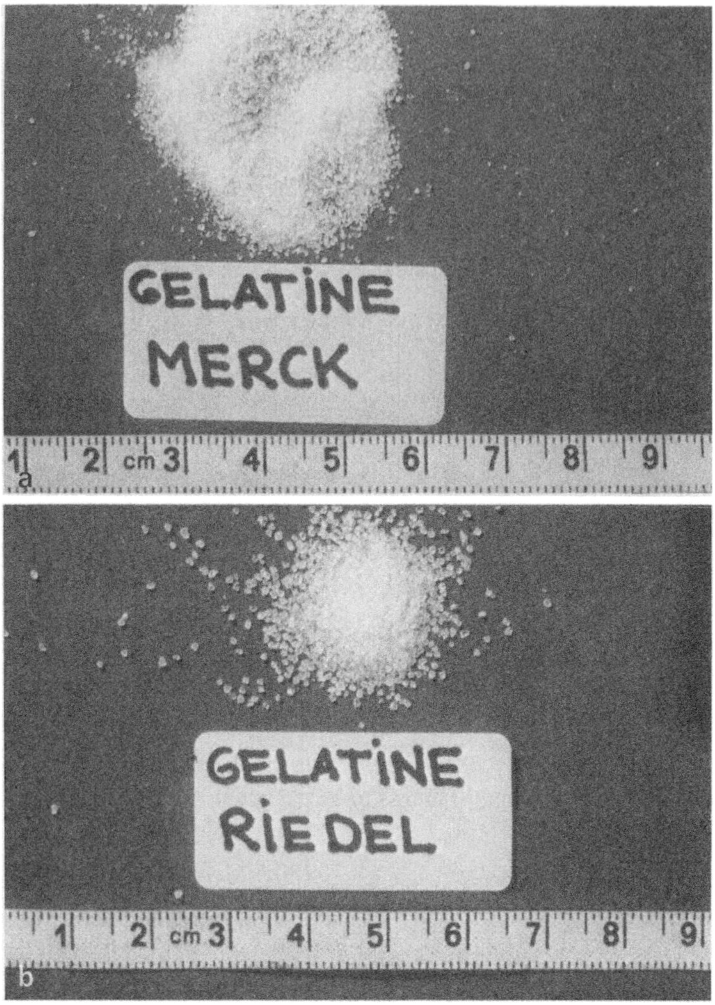

Fig. 5.35 a, b. Gelatin granules before implantation. **a** From Merck (fine). **b** From Riedel (slightly coarser)

exception of a single test after 2 weeks. The artificially introduced bone defect remained clearly visible troughout the entire test series and was still largely unchanged at the end. Thus, **gelatin-filled cavities gave similar results to empty cavities.** As in the empty cavities, the edges of the defect were enhanced by reinforcement of the bone structures; the defect cavity was enclosed in an almost circular manner by strong bony structures.

Twenty gelatin implantations from ten test animals could be used for *quantitative evaluation* (Table 5.13). Three different bone sections per test were made, and the corresponding averages were calculated. The minimum value was 1.1%, the maximum 24.9%; the average for the Merck implants was 7.2%, and that for the Riedel implants was 8.5%. The Wilcoxon pair-difference test was used to test for a statistically significant difference in bone regeneration between Merck implants and Riedel implants, however such a difference could not be demonstrated (Fig. 5.36).

Table 5.13. Quantitative evaluation of bone regeneration under the influence of gelatin particles from Merck (L, left) and Riedel (R, right) after 2–12 weeks

Test number	Test duration (weeks)	Bone formation measured per unit surface area (%)
44L	2	2.7
44R	2	6.9
47L	2	24.9
47R	2	17.5
55L	4	5.3
55R	4	5.5
56L	4	1.2
56R	4	1.6
59L	6	8.0
59R	6	1.1
60L	6	2.1
60R	6	24.3
43L	8	4.3
43R	8	4.2
45L	8	4.7
45R	8	12.5
57L	12	13.8
57R	12	9.0
58L	12	4.8
58R	12	1.9

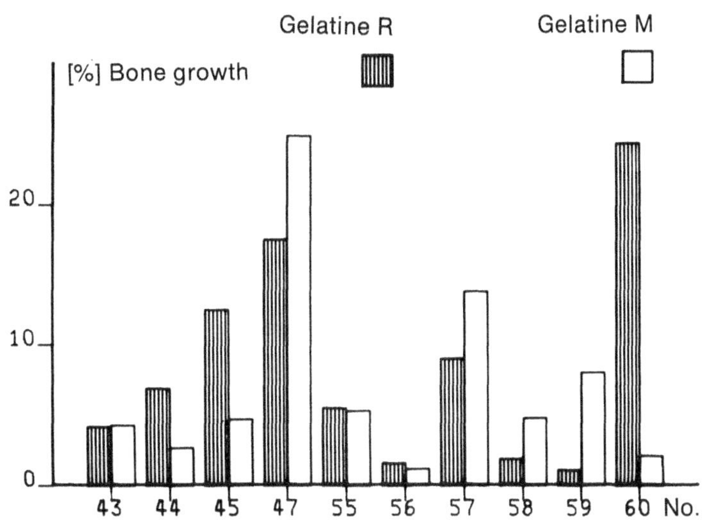

Fig. 5.36. Bone regeneration under the influence of gelatin. There is no statistically significant difference between the two preparations or between either preparation and empty cavities; *R*, Riedel, *M*, Merck

Finally, the Mann-Whitney- U-test was used to establish whether a statistically significant difference existed between gelatin implants and empty cavities. That was also not the case.

The results can be summarised in the conclusion that gelatin preparations do not have a promoting effect on bone growth in comparison to empty cavities (Fig. 5.37). On the other hand, it is remarkable that gelatin does not induce any inflammatory defence reactions at all.

5.4.2.6 Collagen Web with Apatite Powder

Twelve experiments were performed with this implant material. As mentioned previously, this is a commercially prepared, mixed preparation consisting of collagen web and apatite powder (Collapat B), with which Nizard (1981) made his first pilot experiments at the end of his thesis and observed a partially favourable influence on bone regeneration.

The *histological picture* after *6 days* showed that the implant was filled with blood and mostly well preserved. The fine dispersion of powdery apatite could not be clearly discerned in the histological slide, but was clearly visible finely distributed over the entire defect cavity in microradiographs due to the high contrast in the X-ray picture. After *11 days,* some residual implant was still recognisable, but some of it had already been degraded; the defect cavity was filled with the remaining implant and with loose granulation tissue. Peripheral connective tissue structures could be seen, but practically no new bone formation had yet occurred.

After *2 weeks,* peripheral new fibrous bone was seen only very sporadically. The defect cavity was filled with granulation tissue, and the remaining implant had been degraded. In one of the 2-week experiments, about half of the defect cavity was interspersed with loose granulation tissue, while the second half still contained haematoma with initial organisation. The second test did not show any significant formation of new bone after 2 weeks either (Figs. 5.38 and 5.39).

After *4 weeks,* marked inflammatory changes in the connective tissue on the surface of the bone structures were found in test no. 3. Intra-operatively, a hydro-arthrosis with synovial thickening due to inflammation had already been noticed in both knee joints; evaluation of this experiment, therefore, does not seem appropriate, because the inflammatory changes obviously existed before the operation. In the other experiments, *peripheral new bone formation* could be seen after 4 weeks, but most of the defect cavity was interspersed with connective tissue containing many blood vessels. The new bone structures showed massive numbers of osteoblasts and broad osteoid seams. Active bone regeneration was obviously in progress here (Figs. 5.40 and 5.41).

After *6 weeks,* the defect cavity in one of the tests was largely interspersed with new bone trabeculae still exhibiting few osteoblast seams. Some of the gaps in the defect cavity still contained connective tissue; in some gaps normal bone marrow had regenerated. In the second test, the defect cavity was also considerably smaller after 6 weeks due to bone regeneration, but a *large residual defect* still existed.

After *8 weeks,* normal bone marrow had formed again in the defect cavity. The defect cavity had become smaller and stronger due to peripheral formation of new bone, but the *central bulk of the defect was still free of bone* (Fig. 5.42).

After *8 months* the bone defect could no longer be detected with certitude, but a relatively large sector of the epiphysis showed bone deficiency, probably where the defect was located.

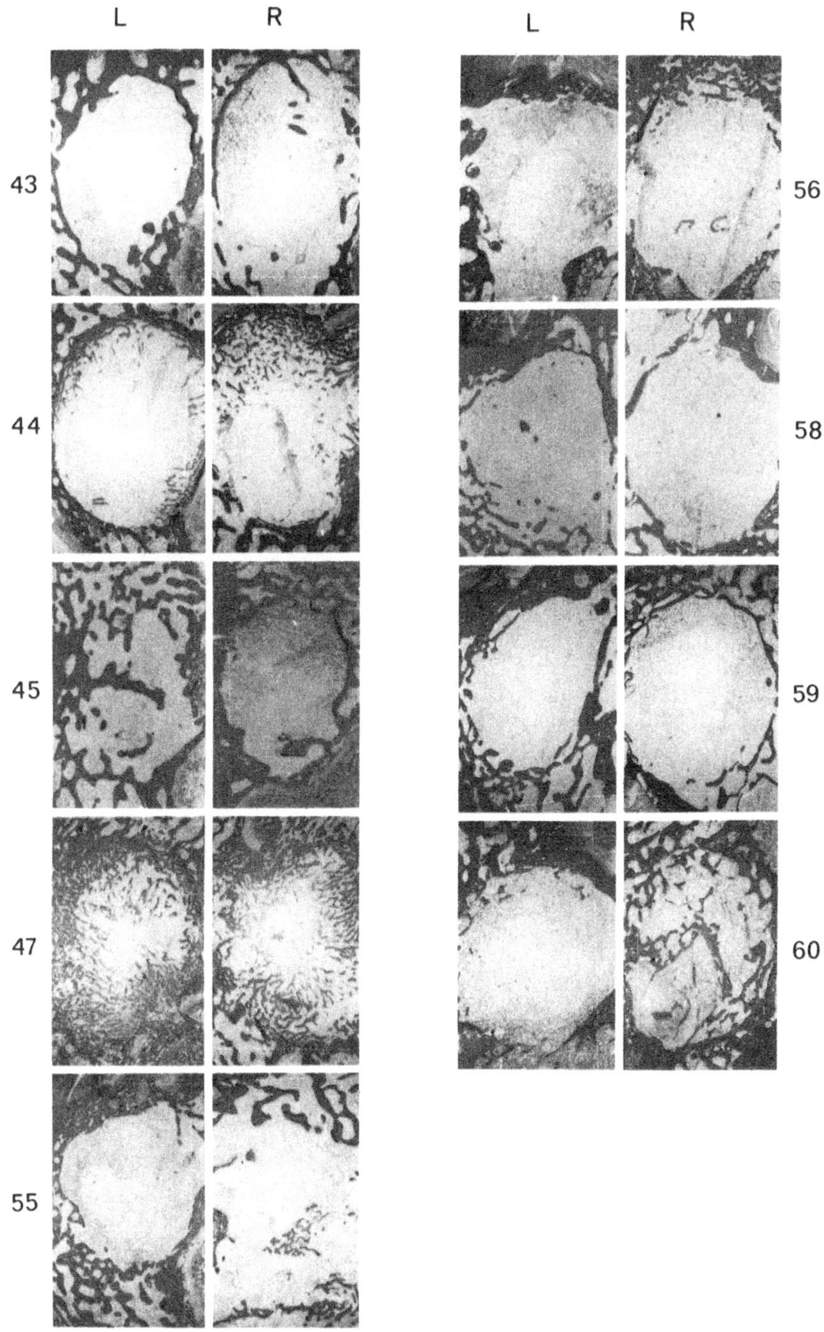

Fig. 5.37. Survey photographs of the preparations with gelatin implantation, showing little, if any, bone regeneration at 2–12 weeks and 8 months; *L,* Merck; *R,* Riedel. The *test number* ist shown next to the *photograph* (MG) × 4

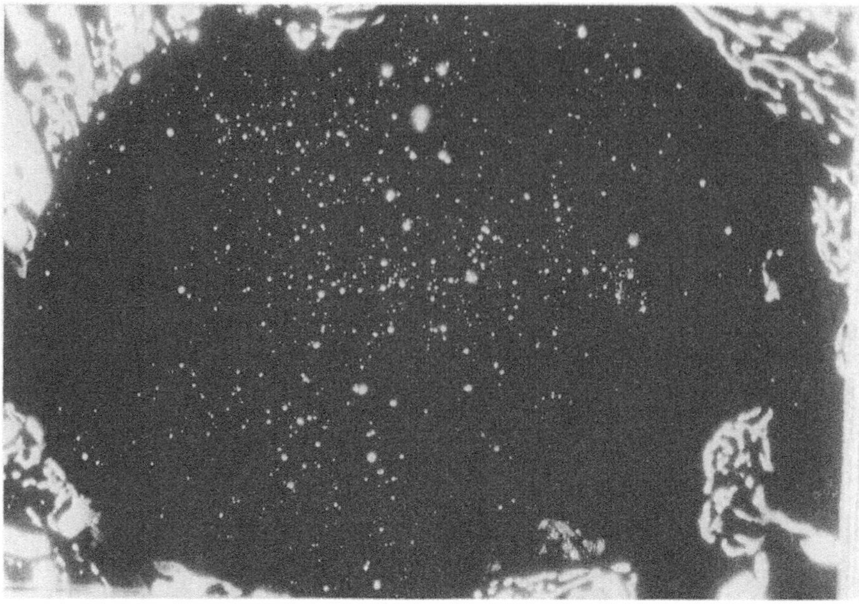

Fig. 5.38. Microradiograph showing fine dispersion of the fine, radio-opaque, powdery apatite particles, but there is no bone regeneration. The effect of the apatite powder is obviously insufficient in this application. (Test 9 right, Collapat B, 2 weeks) × 15

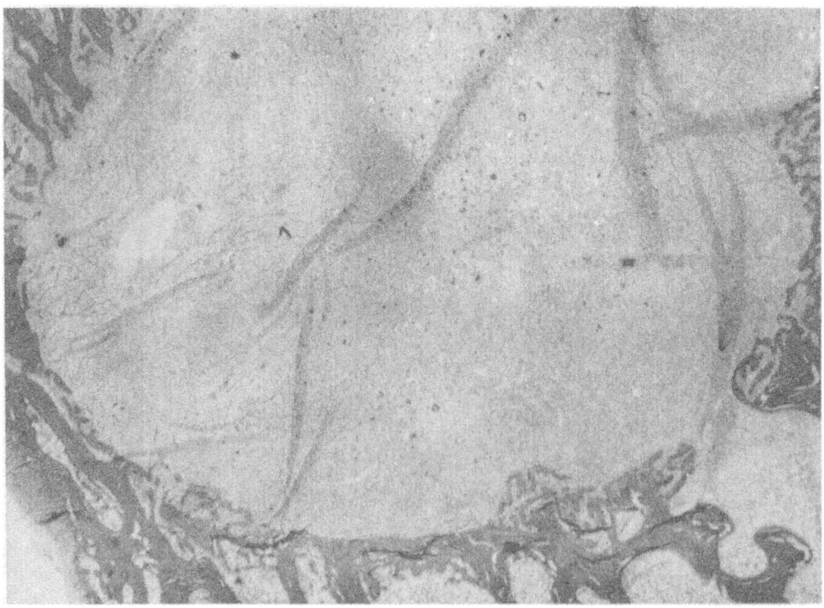

Fig. 5.39. Histological section corresponding to Fig. 5.40. (MG), × 15

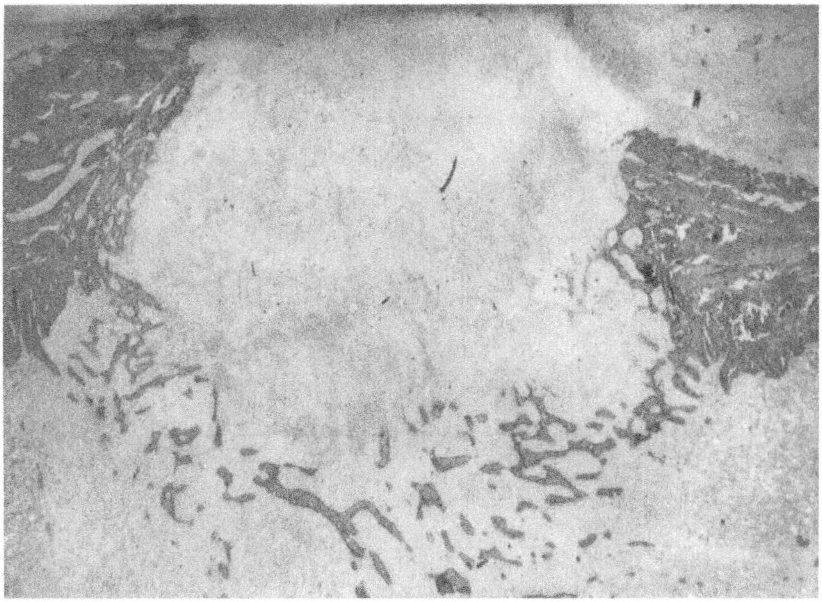

Fig. 5.40. Slight peripheral bone regeneration. (Test 10 right, Collapat B, 4 weeks) MG, × 15

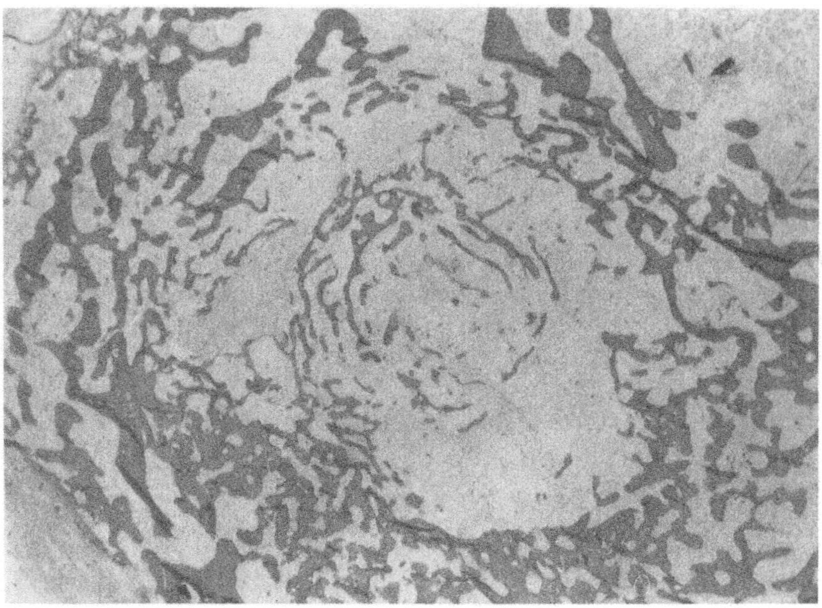

Fig. 5.41. A single test (5 right at 4 weeks) showing marked bone regeneration with Collapat B. On the whole, however, the Collapat B series is not very convincing. MG, × 15

Collapat B

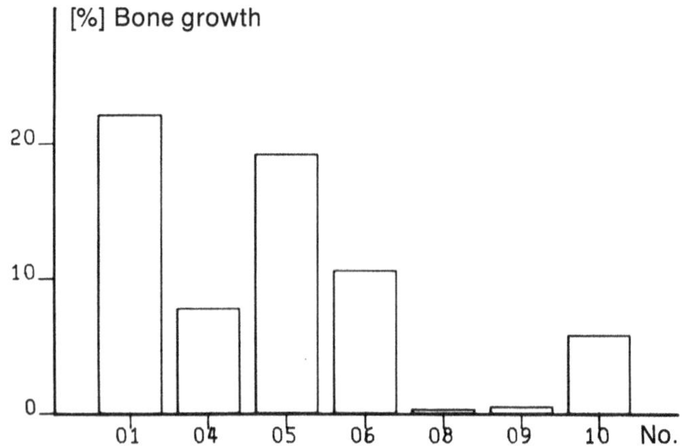

Fig. 5.42. Bone regeneration with Collapat B. In the seven tests evaluated, no significant difference in comparison to empty cavities was found

The apatite powder was no longer visible by *microradiography* after 6 weeks, and sometimes as early as 4 weeks. It had obviously been resorbed by this time.

From our own experiments, seven tests between 2 and 8 weeks could be evaluated (Table 5.14). The relative surface areas of regenerated bone were 0.3% at a minimum and 22.1% at a maximum, with an average of 9.4%. Bone regeneration was therefore only *slightly better* than in the empty cavities. Apparently, the promoting effect of apatite powder on bone regeneration reported in some cases by Nizard (1981) was *not generally effective enough* in this application. Probably, the concentration and the quantity of apatite powder used were too low (Fig. 5.43).

Statistical comparison of the results obtained after implantation of this Collapat B preparation with the results obtained for empty cavities did not show a significant difference at a confidence level of $P = 0.1$ in the Mann-Whitney U-test. It is possible that

Table 5.14. Relative surface area of regenerated bone in the defect cavity under the influence of collagen web with apatite powder (Collapat B) between 2 and 8 weeks

Test number	Test period (weeks)	Bone regeneration per measured area (%)
8R	2	0.3
9R	2	0.5
5R	4	19.2
10R	4	5.8
1R	6	22.1
4R	8	7.8
6R	8	10.6

R, right

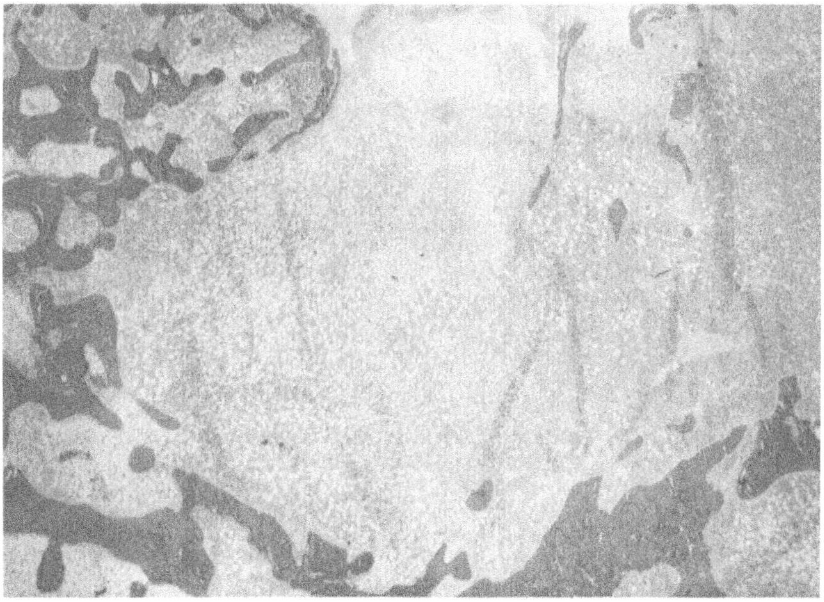

Fig. 5.43. Only slight peripheral bone regeneration. (Test 4 right, Collapat B, 8 weeks) MG, × 15

a statistically significant difference would arise with a larger number of tests, although the present data already suggest that such a difference would certainly be quite small. Since we were able to obtain considerably better results with improved implantation materials, as will be explained further on, we decided, for reasons of animal welfare, not to expand the series with further testing of this implantation material.

5.4.2.7 Ceramised Apatite Granules (Apagran)

Pure apatite granules, i.e. without carrier, were implanted in 12 tests (Fig. 5.44). First of all, we have to point out that we experienced considerable difficulties with the operating technique when implanting ceramised apatite granules with an *average size of approx. 250 μm.* Since these granules were incorporated in loose form without a carrier, it was very difficult to fill the defect cavities in the presence of bleeding, because the granules were *washed out* by the blood stream. Consequently, the histological preparation showed large variations in the degree to which the cavities had been filled with apatite granules. Also, *sedimentation* of the granules proves to be a problem, so that the distribution of the granules in the defect cavity is very irregular. Therefore, from a surgical viewpoint, this implantation material is *not very suitable* in this form.

In the test after *6 days,* the apatite granules had sedimented *only at the edge* of the defect. Most of the defect cavity did not contain any apatite particles, and was occupied by a haematoma with early organisation. Peripheral granulation tissue could already be detected. The surface of the apatite granules was covered with a *delicate layer of cells,* which had settled directly on the apatite granule in an epithelioid manner. These cells were bulb-shaped, but could not be identified with certainty as osteoblasts; they may have been pre-osteoblasts. Other sectors showed an amorphous seam, on the surface of

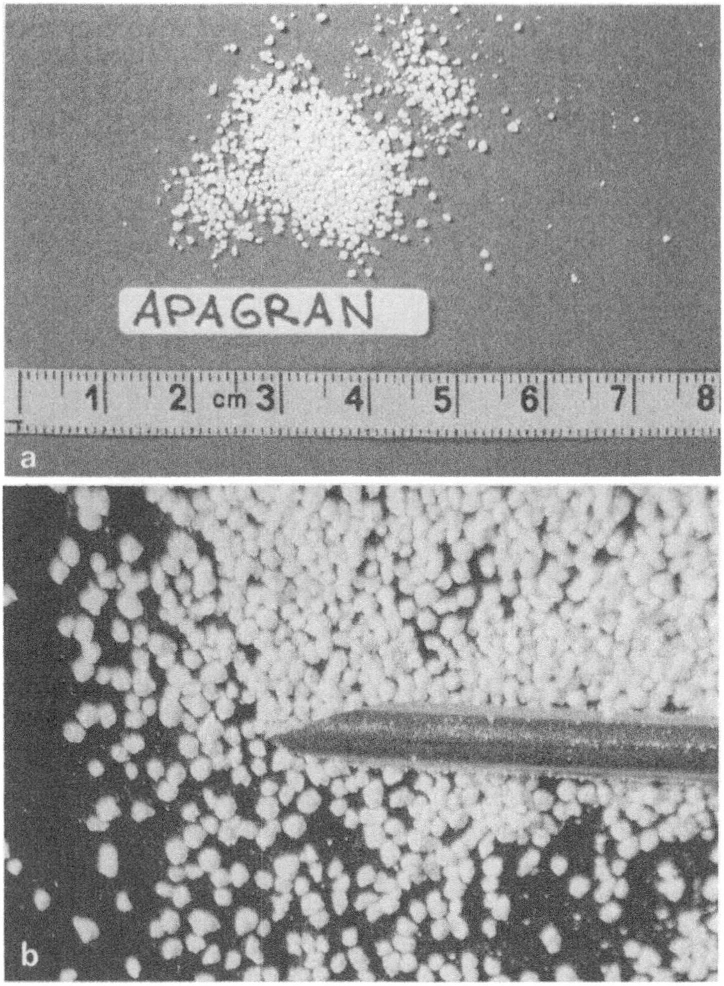

Fig. 5.44a, b. Apagran (hydroyapatite ceramic material in the form of fine granules). These granules were isolated in several sizes (50–500 μm), or tested after embedding in a collagen web (Collapat D and Collapat E)

the apatite granules, which took on a pale pink colour with Masson-Goldner staining. The irregular distribution of the apatite granules in the defect cavity was also apparent in subsequent sections.

After *11 days,* the peripheral apatite granules were *already surrounded by regenerated bone,* and there was no separating interface layer between the apatite granules and the new bone. At this time, *osteoblasts* could be detected directly on the surface of the apatite granules, which were embedded in previously mineralised bone tissue and would eventually develop into osteocytes. In other sectors, large numbers of osteocytes were found directly on the surface of the apatite granules and on the surface of the regenerated bone structures. Almost no osteoid seams were visible, which leads to the conclusion that *newly formed osteoids are immediately mineralised.*

In one test after *2 weeks,* no apatite granules at all were visible; they had obviously been washed out, and there was no bone regeneration in the defect cavity. On the other hand, in the second 2-week test there was *massive* bone regeneration in direct contact with the apatite granules. In some cases, the peripheral apatite granules had already been completely surrounded by bone. In other cases there was obviously a massive line-up of osteoblasts and pre-osteoblasts occurring on the surface of the apatite granules (Figs. 5.45 and 5.46).

Everywhere, many blood vessels and sometimes loose connective tissue were seen. **Massive bone regeneration, which had not been observed in any of the implants described so far** was occurring (Figs. 5.47–5.51).

After *4 weeks,* bone regeneration was observed on the surface of almost all the apatite granules, and almost exclusively there. It was apparent that bone regeneration was occurring in connection with, and influenced by, the apatite granules (Figs. 5.52 and 5.53).

The *irregular distribution of the apatite granules over the defect cavity* explains the observation that *no bone regeneration occurred in the apatite-free zones* of these sections. The apatite granules appeared to be somewhat too large, so that there was a certain disparity between their size and the bone regeneration occurring on their surface.

After *6 weeks,* the apatite granules were firmly embedded, like a crystallisation centre, in regenerated bone. The individual fibrous bone trabeculae now started to interconnect with each other, thereby forming a reinforced bony structure within the defect. On the other hand, large zones containing no apatite were also present, and these exhibited almost no bone. The bone trabeculae in the defect cavities seemed more mature, and some of them had a laminar structure (Fig. 5.54).

After *8 months,* the apatite granules were still clearly discernible, and continued to be encompassed by regenerated bone. Some of the apatite granules had crumbled away during the cutting process. It is, however, remarkable that the zone of direct contact with the regenerated bone often remains intact. One has the impression that *the bond between the apatite granule and the regenerated bone is so strong* that the granule itself, rather than the bond between its surface and the regenerated bone, will be torn apart.

In the test after 8 months, the defect cavity was homogeneously filled with apatite granules. The observation described earlier, that apatite granules with a size of 250 μm are too large and take up too much space, is particularly evident in Fig. 5.57.

Importantly, in all the experiments with Apagran, over the entire test period, *no inflammatory or other defensive reactions at all* were observed. The implant was obviously not only well tolerated, but *stimulates bone regeneration directly on its surface without any separating layer of connective tissue* (Figs. 5.56–5.58).

Some problems were encountered with the histological technique used in this test series, in that some of the sections were technically unsatisfactory: wrinkle-formation and bone ruptures were frequent. The blocks embedded in methylmethacrylate were stored for 3 months before the sections were cut. This probably led to further hardening of the blocks, which then caused problems when the micro-sections were prepared. Later, we sectioned the blocks immediately after embedding, and modified the cutting technique, as described earlier, thereby solving this problem in the later experimental series. Hard ceramised apatite granules, which are partly embedded in soft tissue, call for particular care when performing undecalcified bone histology. In view of these problems, we did *not* make a *quantitative evaluation* of these sections, because we considered

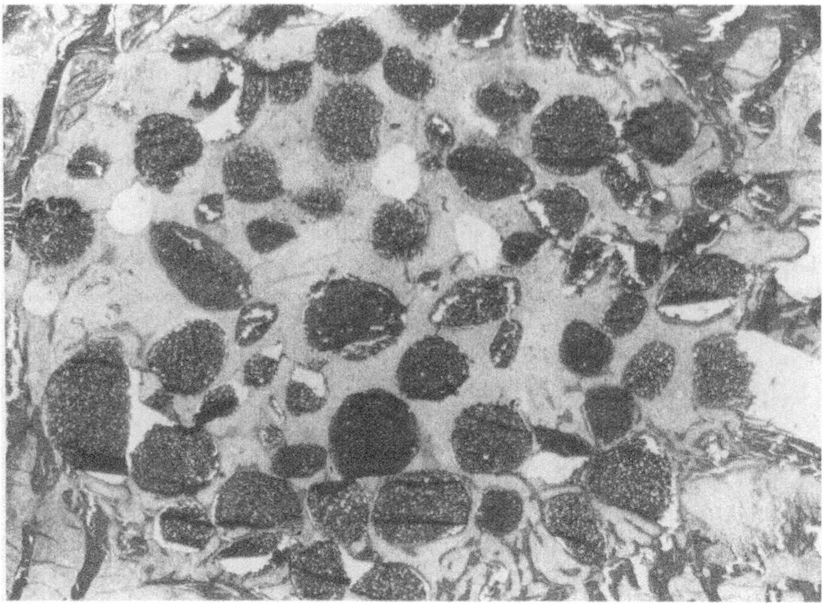

Fig. 5.45. Initial peripheral bone regeneration around the hydroxyapatite granules. (Test 8 left, Apagran, 2 weeks) MG, × 15

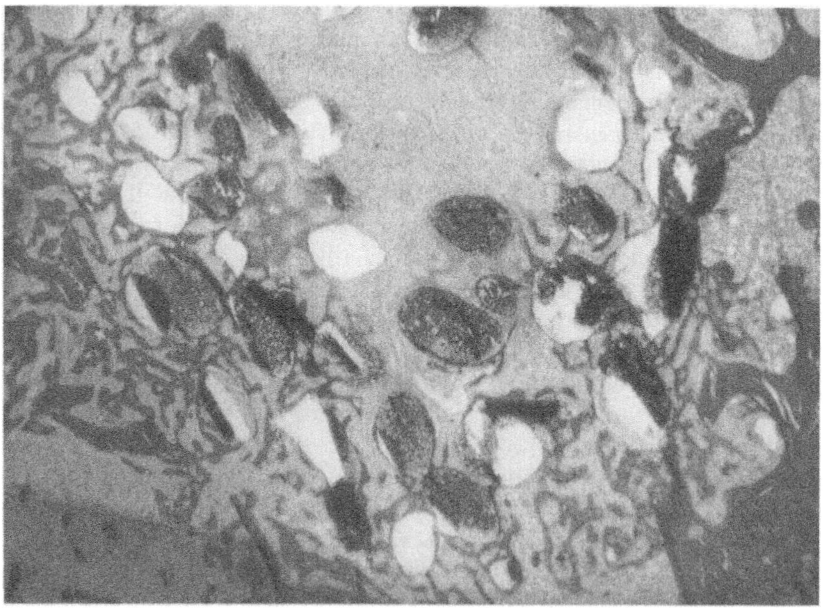

Fig. 5.46. Intensive bone regeneration progressing centripetally between the hydroxyapatite granules. Bone regeneration can be seen in direct contact with the implanted particles. (Test 9 left, Apagran, 2 weeks) × 18

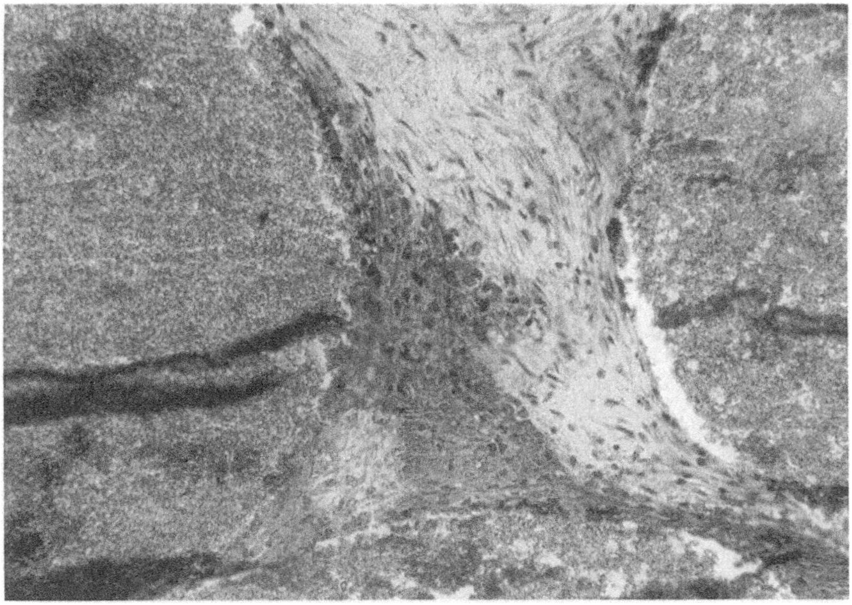

Fig. 5.47. Early phase of bone regeneration on hydroxyapatite (HA) granules (*left, right, below*). Osteoblasts (*black*) line up directly against the HA surface, adjacent to previously mineralised bone (*dark grey*). (Test 8 left, Apagran, 2 weeks) MG, × 150

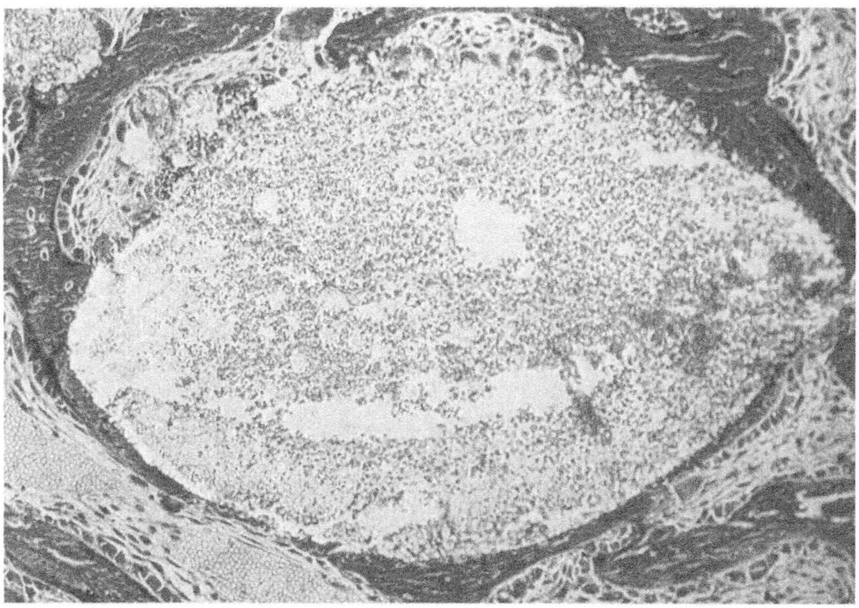

Fig. 5.48. The HA granules are surrounded by regenerated bone indicating intensive bone regeneration. The implant obviously favours bone deposition. × 150

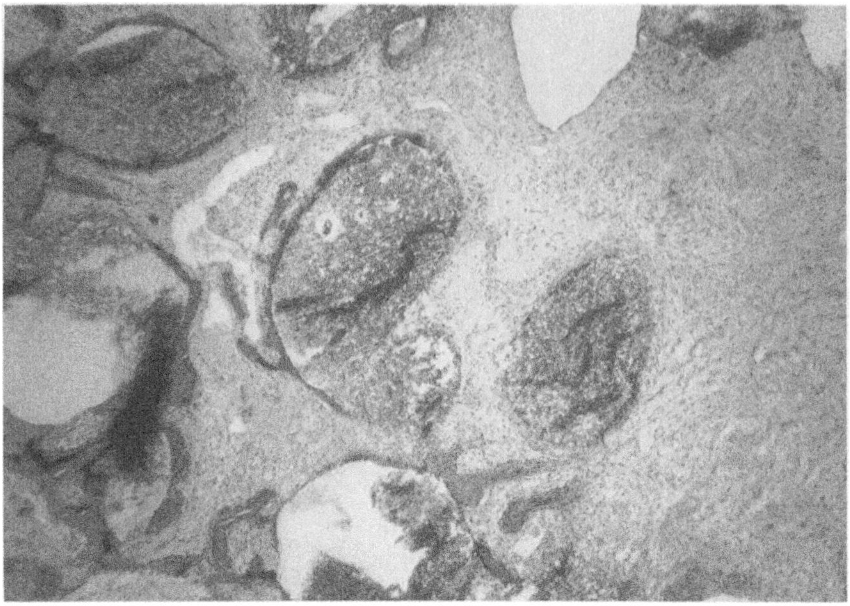

Fig. 5.49. Early bone regeneration directly on the surface of the apatite granules; the section includes many blood vessels. (Test 9 left, Apagran, 2 weeks) × 40

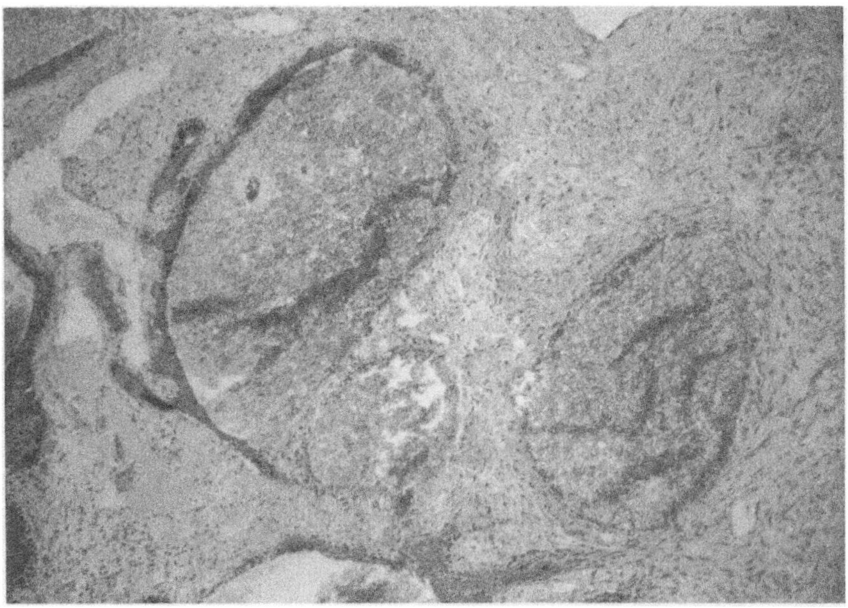

Fig. 5.50. No separating layer of connective tissue exists between bone and implant. (Enlarged sector of Fig. 5.49) × 70

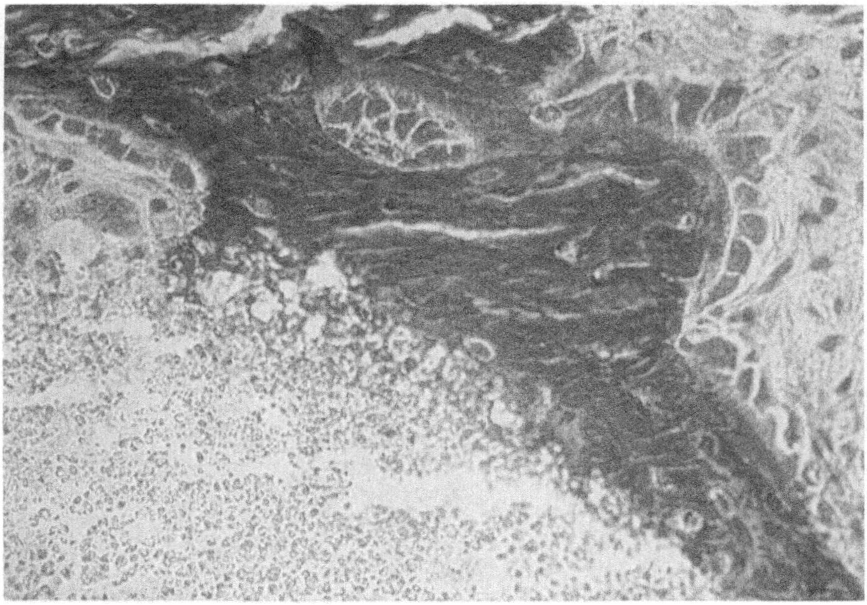

Fig. 5.51. Regenerated bone (*dark*) in intimate contact with hydroxyapatite (*below left*). (Test 9 left, Apagran, 2 weeks) × 300

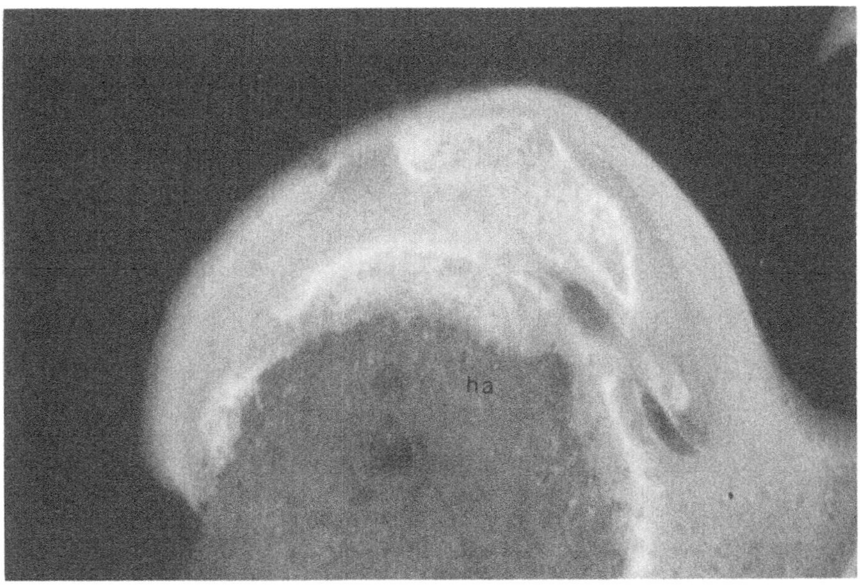

Fig. 5.52. Incorporation of fluorescent dyes into regenerated bone surrounding the hydroxyapatite. (Test 5 left, Apagran, 4 weeks) Fluorescence staining, × 150

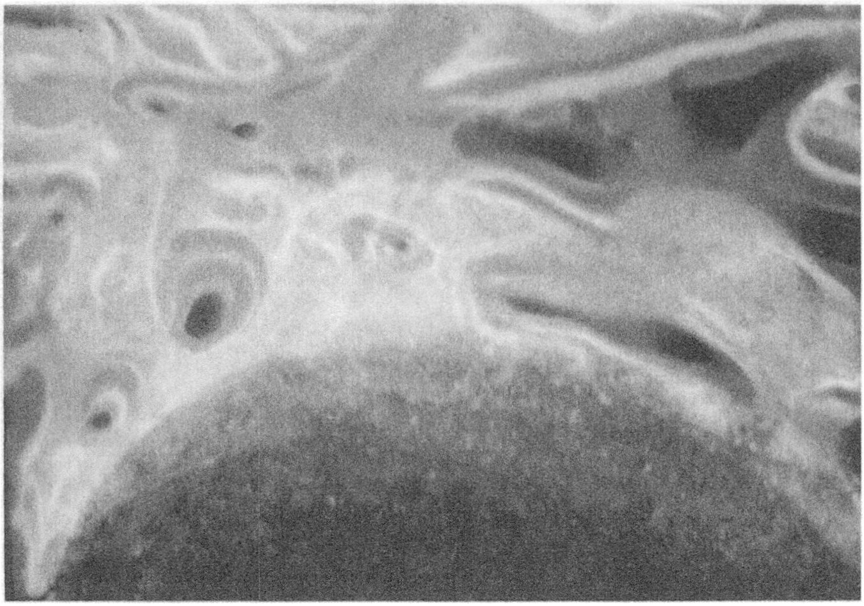

Fig. 5.53. Similar findings to those in Fig. 5.52, in another sector

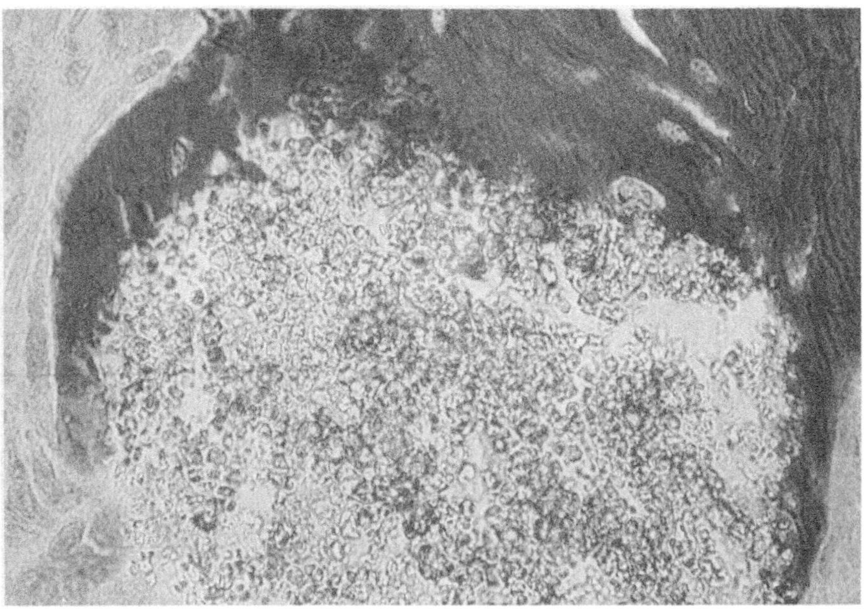

Fig. 5.54. After 6 weeks, basically the same findings as in Fig. 5.51

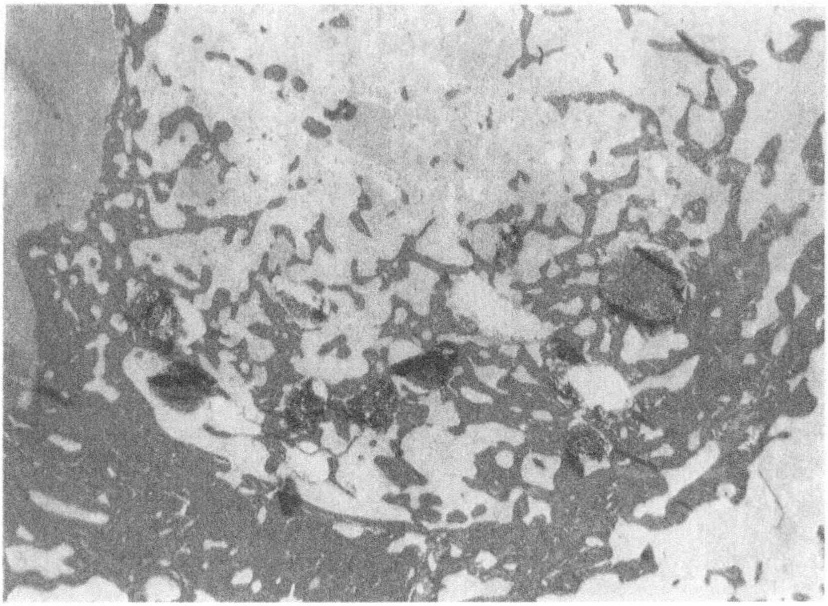

Fig. 5.55. Irregular filling of the drilled cavity due to sedimentation and washing by blood. Bone regeneration around the hydroxyapatite granules. (Test 1 left, Apagran, 6 weeks) MG, × 15

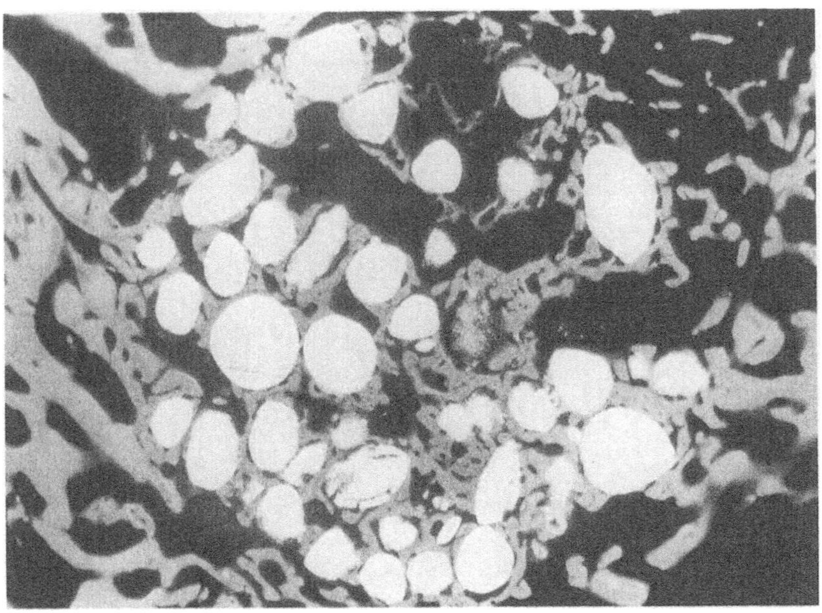

Fig. 5.56. The radio-opaque hydroxyapatite particles (*white*) are completely surrounded by regenerated bone. (Test 1 left, Apagran, 6 weeks, microradiograph) × 15

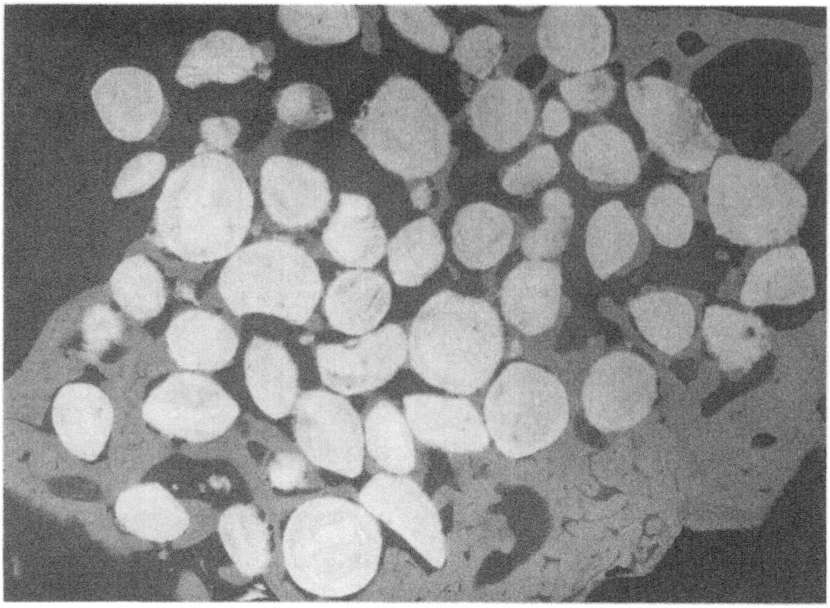

Fig. 5.57. The network between hydroxyapatite particles and regenerated bone persists for a long time. The granules are integrated into the regenerated bone. (Test 7 left, Apagran, 8 months, microradiograph) × 15

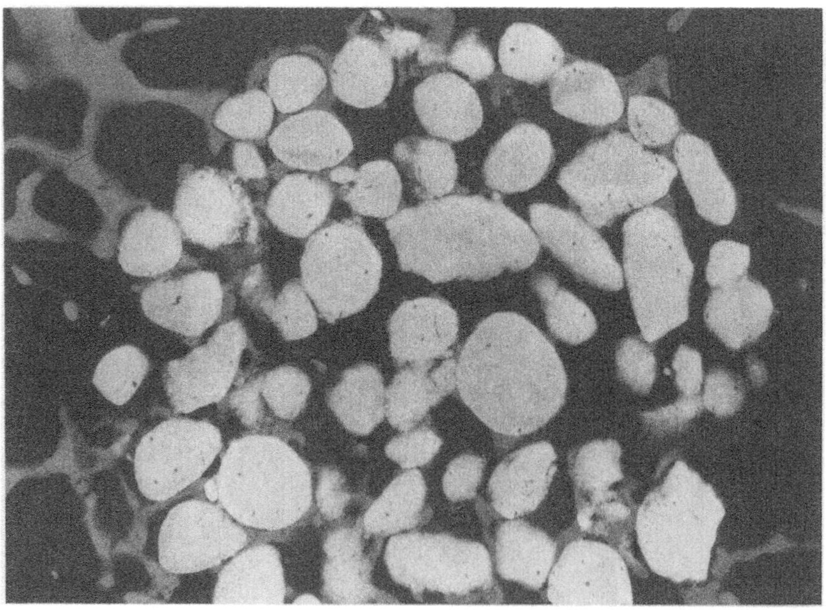

Fig. 5.58. Although the hydroxyapatite granules are integrated into the bone matrix everywhere, they appear too large and take up too much space. It seems desirable to reduce the size of the granules to free more space for the bone. (Test 6 left, Apagran, 8 weeks, microradiograph) × 15

that the error possibilities due to wrinkles, ruptures of the bone and partially dissolved bone substance were too great.

After observing the obvious *stimulation* of bone regeneration by *ceramised apatite granules* and the unsatisfactory regenerative capacity with the use of powdery apatite, ceramised apatite granules (embedded in collagen web and of smaller size) were used in subsequent experiments, so that quantitative evaluation was possible later.

Not all implants of ceramised apatite granules were located ideally in the epiphysis. Occasionally, an implant found its way into marrow or soft tissue. It was found that in the case of implantations into the femoral canal, bone regeneration also occured on the surface of the apatite granules but was considerably reduced in comparison to implantation into the spongiosa. In the case of pure soft-tissue implantation, however, no significant bone regeneration was found, showing that the particularly favourable stimulating effect of apatite granules on bone regeneration is limited to implantation in *strongly regenerative* stroma.

5.4.2.8 Collagen Web with Ceramised Apatite Granules (Collapat D)

To solve the problems encountered during implantation of ceramised apatite granules (washing out of the implantation site, post-operative sedimentation, overly large particles) we developed our system further, and reduced the particle size of the apatite granules to 100–150 μm. We had recource to the concept of multi-centric regeneration, taking into consideration the results obtained by Nizard (1981), and used the collagen web as carrier for the fine apatite granulese. Fine apatite granules were sintered from the powdery, synthetic hydroxyapatite, and then mixed industrially in a weight ratio of apatite to collagen of 5:1 in the wet phase with collagen web.

With this implantation material, called Collapat D, we first ran a series of six pilot experiments (Fig. 5.59). The results obtained were quite surprising. The application of this implant was of course much simpler than that of loose apatite granules, especially since the collagen web used as the carrier had some haemostatic effect, probably by tamponnage.

Histology now showed predominantly homogeneous dispersion throughout the defect cavity. After only *2 weeks*, the *granules were walled in with bone,* and since the numerous small apatite granules offer a large number of crystallisation centres for bone regeneration, which are also closer together, *complete ossification of the defect cavity was observed after only 2 weeks* in one of the tests. Large numbers of osteoblasts were present everywhere, bone regeneration had progressed further according to the scheme described in Sect. 5.4.2.7. Bone regeneration occurred *directly on the surface of the apatite granules, and no inflammatory defensive reactions at all* were manifest (Figs. 5.60 and 5.61).

After *4 weeks,* these regenerated bone structures appeared considerably wider, were linked together, and formed a strong bony framework extending throughout the entire defect. The small apatite granules seemed to have been *incorporated into the bone,* and would not interfere with subsequent bone remodelling processes. Owing to their homogeneous distribution and small particle size, they also *did not interfere with the formation of blood vessels with in the defect cavity in any way.*

The defect cavities did not always lie exactly with in the distal femoral epiphysis, but sometimes extended into the femoral canal. Bone regeneration was also observed on

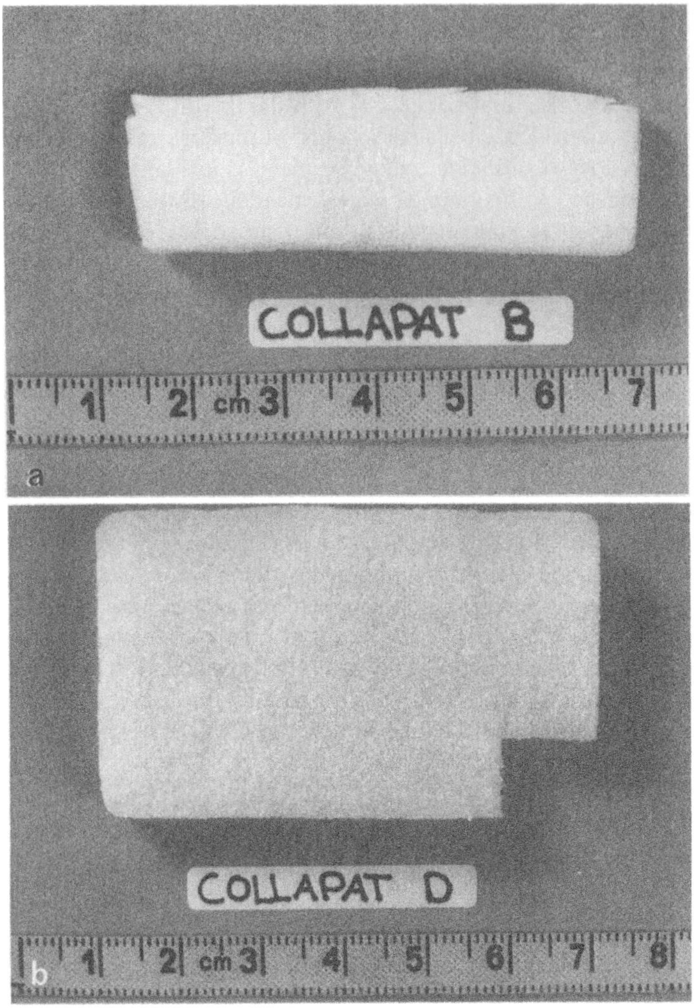

Fig. 5.59 a, b. The ceramised apatite granules in Collapat D (**b**) are macroscopically visible in contrast to the powder in Collapat B (**a**)

apatite granules located in the femoral canal, although to a somewhat lesser extent. In one of the 2-week sections, however, a still-unsatisfactory distribution (irregular, incomplete) of the apatite particles in the defect cavity was found. We interpreted this to mean that the collagen web which we used possibly dissolved too readily and was resorbed too quickly, so that *homogeneous distribution of the heavy apatite ceramic particles was not maintained long enough* (Figs. 5.62 and 5.63).

The difference, in quantity of regenerated bone, between cavities filled with Collapat D and the corresponding empty cavities on the opposite side was impressive. In defect cavities filled with Collapat D, the relative surface area of regenerated bone had a minimum value of 15.1%, a maximum of 25.1% and an average of 19.6%. In the empty cavities there was a minimum of 0.6%, a maximum of 10.9% and 5.0% on average. The

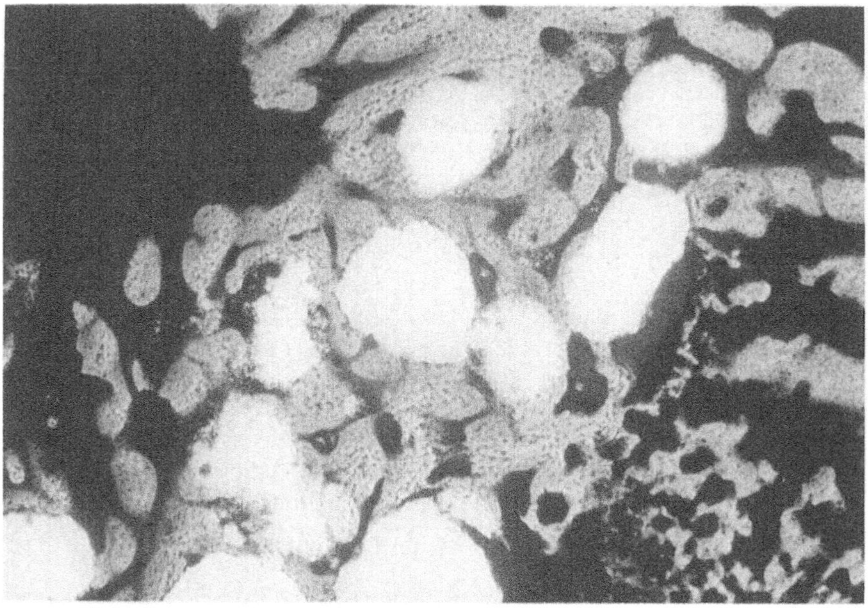

Fig. 5.60. Microradiograph showing bone regeneration (yellow) at the implantation site of the apatite particles (*white*). The marrow cavity is black. (Test 42 left, Collapat D, 4 weeks) × 90

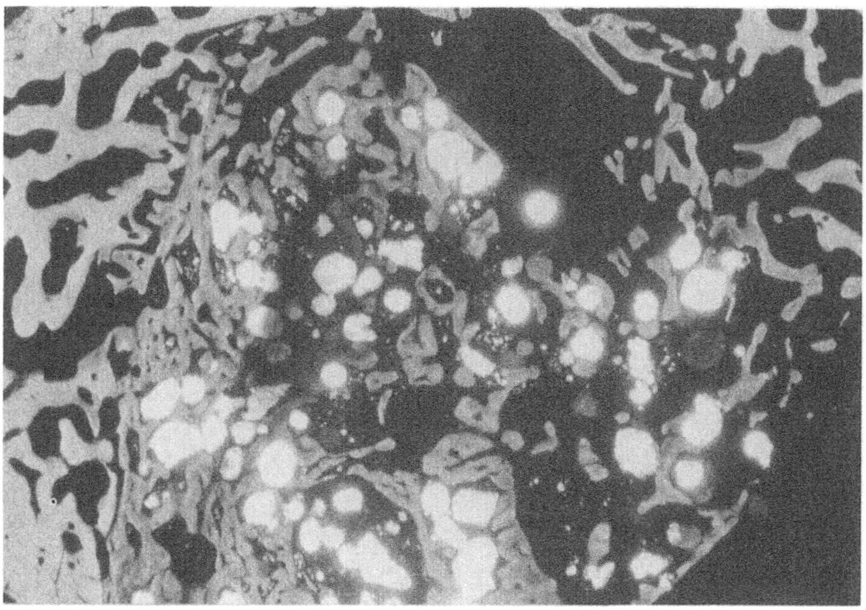

Fig. 5.61. Microradiograph demonstrates that smaller size of hydroxyapatite particles does not adversely affect bone regeneration (*yellow*). On the contrary, a denser bony network is formed. (Test 39 left, Collapat D, 6 weeks). Compare with the empty cavity on the other side in Fig. 5.63. × 15

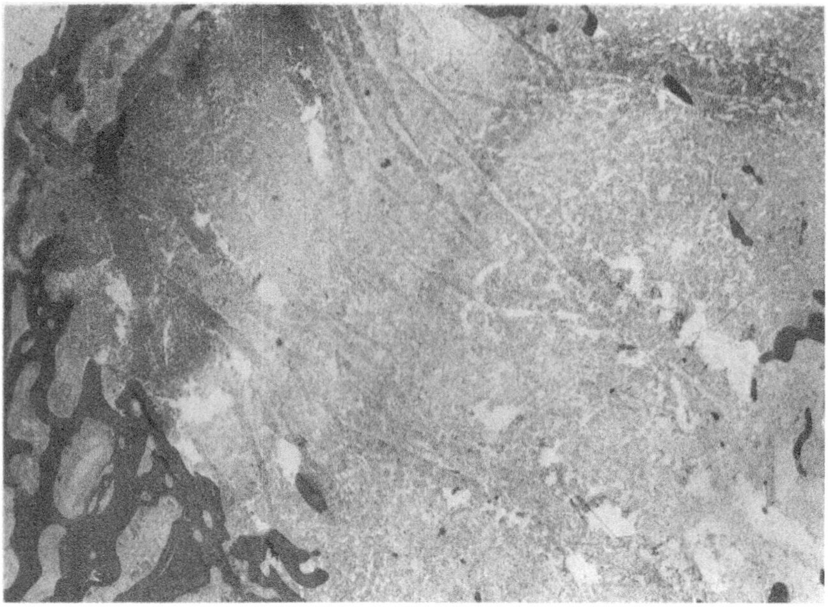

Fig. 5.62. Practically no bone regeneration has occurred. (Test 39 right, empty cavity, 6 weeks) Compare with Fig. 5.61. MG, × 15

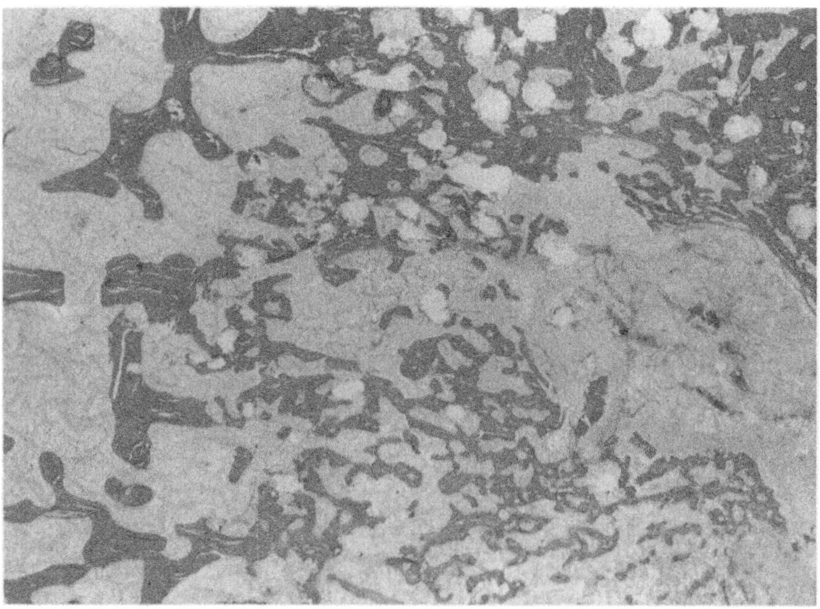

Fig. 5.63. The stimulating effect of hydroxyapatite on bone regeneration is enhanced by reducing the size of the granules (some of which have crumbled away from the slide), since additional space for bone growth is created. (Test 42 left, Collapat D, 4 weeks). The contrast to the empty cavity on the opposite side is impressive (compare with Fig. 5.64). MG, × 25

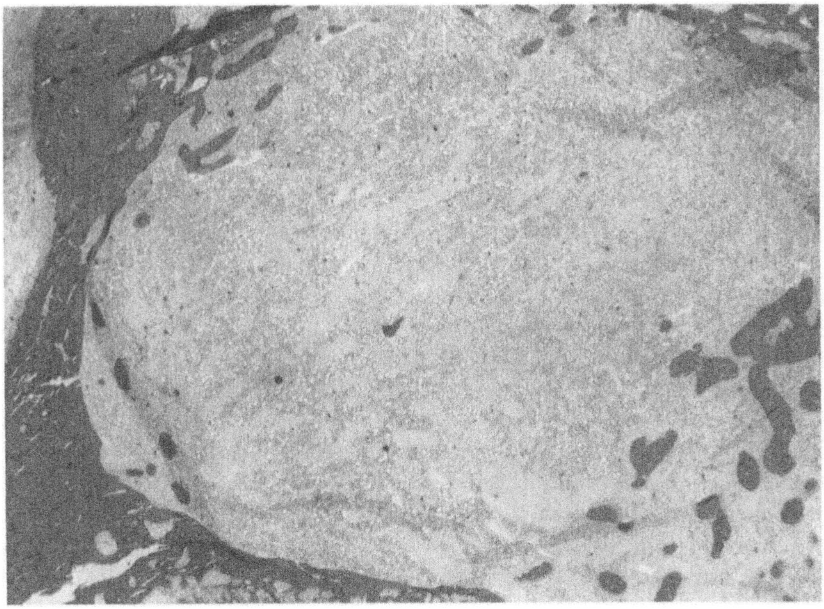

Fig. 5.64. Test 42 right (empty cavity), × 15

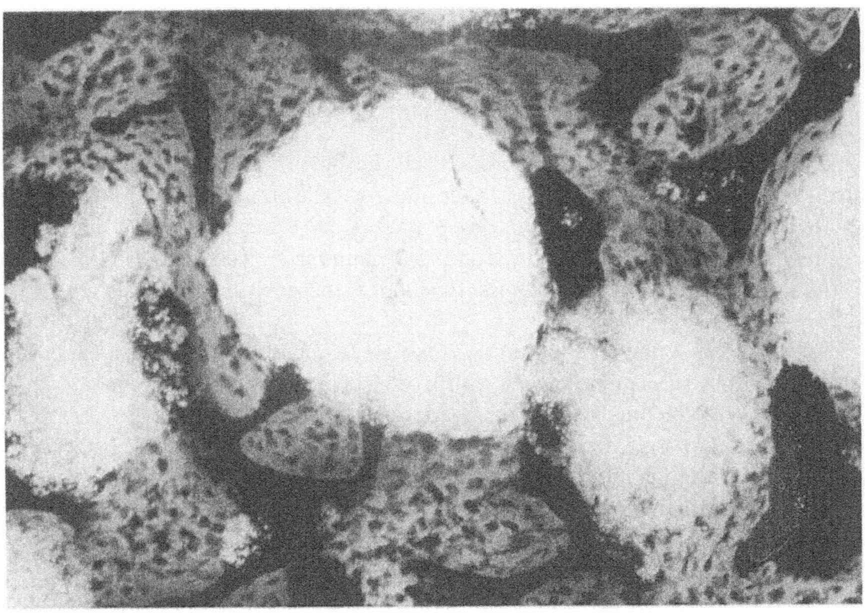

Fig. 5.65. Enlarged sector from Fig. 5.60. (Test 42 left, Collapat D, 4 weeks). Hydroxyapatite granules and bone form a tight bond. × 250

rate of bone regeneration with Collapat D was therefore about *four times higher than in empty cavities,* a result which we never even approached with any of the bone-replacement materials mentioned earlier. The difference was impressive enough, but could not be confirmed statistically in this small test series, particularly since only four tests fulfilled the technical requirements for quantitative evaluation (Figs. 5.63 and 5.64).

5.4.2.9 Cross-linked Collagen Web with Small Ceramised Apatite Granules (Collapat E)
Since some irregularities of distribution were still encountered in the previous test series, the collagen web used as a carrier for the fine apatite ceramic particles was subjected to a secondary cross-linking process in order to obtain additional *structural stabilisation,* and then *mixed industrially in the wet phase* in a weight ratio of apatite to collagen of 5:1 (Figs. 5.66 and 5.67). Since this implantation material showed by far the best stimulating effect on bone regeneration of all bone-replacement materials we tested in our experiments, we performed two test series with this material for quantitative statistical evaluation *using the pair-difference test versus empty cavities* on the one hand and *versus autogenic spongiosa transplants* on the other.

Experiments were evaluated after the following time periods: 1, 2, 3, 4, 6, 8 and 12 weeks and after 8 months, a total of 28 implantations on 28 rabbits. Some of the test results have already been published (Katthagen and Mittelmeier 1984) (Fig. 5.68).

After *1 week,* the defect cavity appeared to be homogeneously filled with dispersed apatite ceramic particles. The collagen web, which acts as carrier, was permeated by haematoma; peripheral proliferation of blood vessels was beginning. In a further test after only 1 week, peripheral regenerated bone was found as well as a large number of mesenchymal cells, which line up directly on the surfaces of the apatite granules.

After *2 weeks,* new blood vessels which had grown in towards the centre were seen throughout the defect cavity, as well as remnants of the haematoma, which was undergoing organisation. In one of the 2-week tests, half of the bone defect was filled with a *tight meshwork of regenerated fibrous bone.* Bone regeneration directly on the surfaces of the apatite granules was also found comparable with Apagran and Collapat D (Figs. 5.69–5.71).

In the further course of the experiment, the meshwork of fibrous bone became denser, the bone trabeculae broader, the surface area over the bone defect larger, and *almost the entire defect cavity was filled with regenerated bone.* When comparing the bone defect with adjacent intact bone structures one could gain the impression that the *bone network within the defect area was even denser than that in the surrounding region* (Figs. 5.72 and 5.73).

After *4 weeks,* bone regeneration was complete. *The entire defect was filled with bone, and completely structured,* again with a denser bone framework than in the intact surroundings. Not only was bone regeneration directed towards the surfaces of the apatite particles, a phenomenon which Burchardt (1983) described as osteoconduction (as opposed to induction) but what must be described as *massive stimulation of osteoregeneration as a whole, including the gaps* occurred. *Primary bone formation* takes place, and not subsequent ossification of intermediary connective tissue as is the case for callous formation. Also, this **osteoconduction does not proceed via osteoclastic resorption of transplanted bone tissue, but rather through immediate primary stimulation of new bone formation in the ingrowing granulation tissue.**

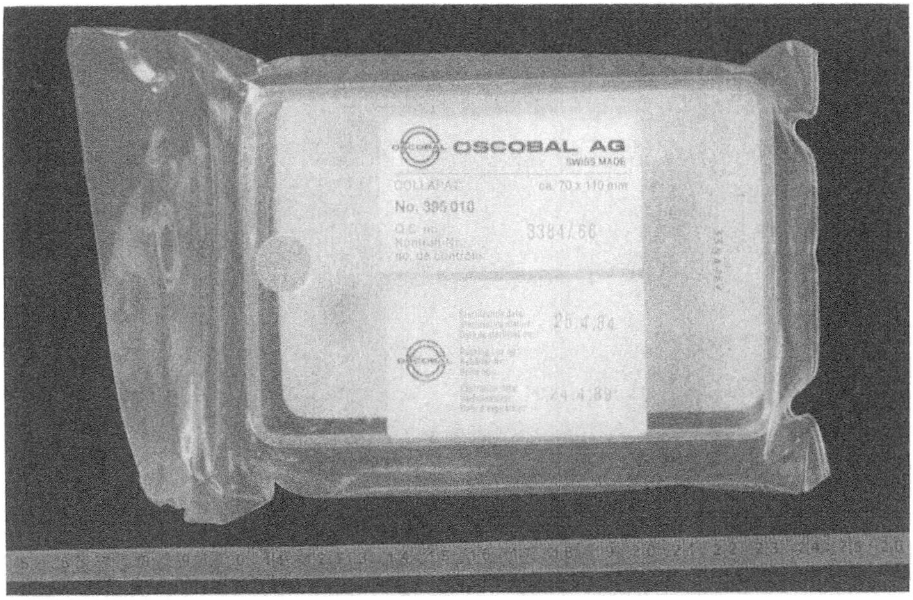

Fig. 5.66. The final development product Collapat E is supplied by Oscobal AG under the trade-name Collapat, and is packaged in welded plastic film and radiation-sterilised

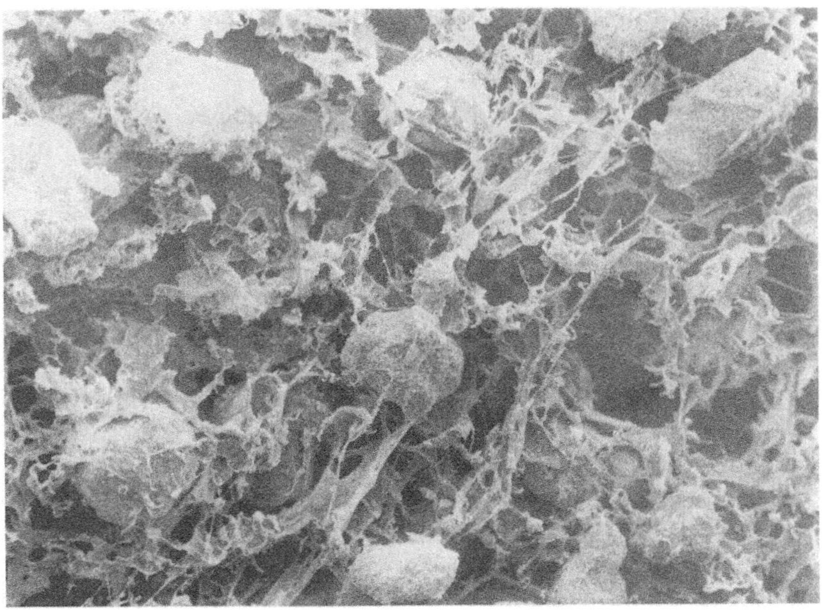

Fig. 5.67. In the scanning electron micrograph of Collapat, the fine meshwork of the collagen web used as carrier substance and the finely dispersed distribution of the ceramised apatite granules are clearly visible

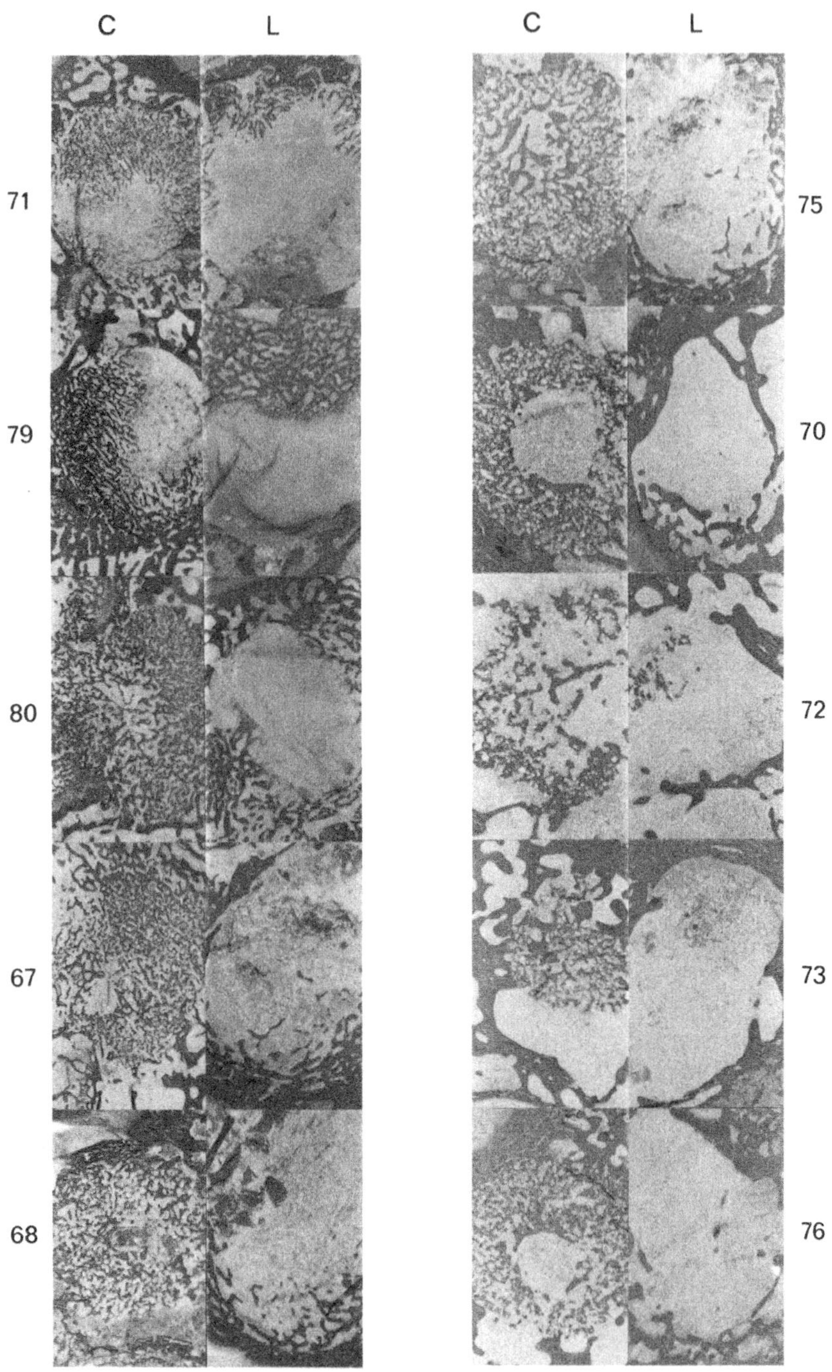

Fig. 5.68. Series of survey photographs, showing predominantly complete bone regeneration in cavities filled with Collapat E. There has been slight and incomplete filling of the defect for empty cavities; *C,* Collapat E; *L,* empty cavity. (Test number *next to the photograph,* 2–12 weeks) MG, × 4

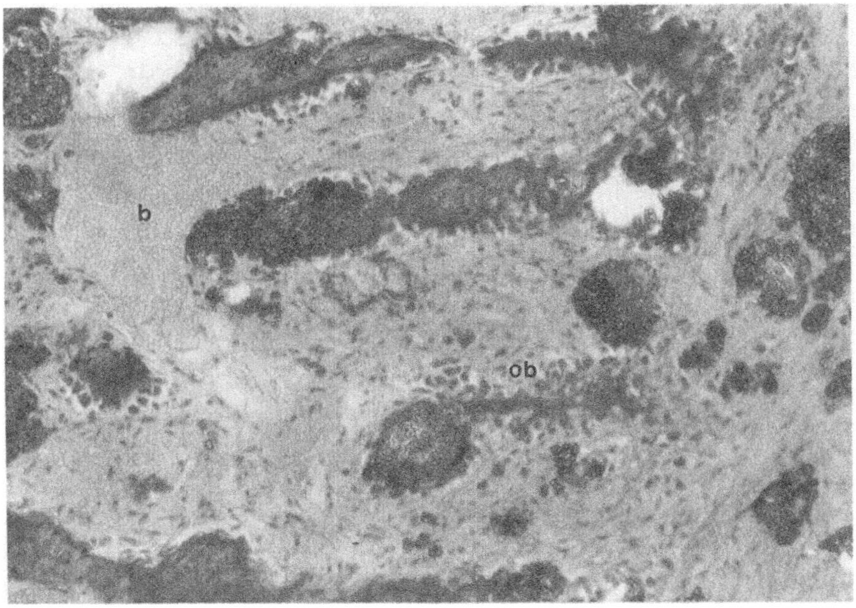

Fig. 5.69. Early phase of bone regeneration on the surface of HA granules (*grey-granular*). Osteoblasts (*ob*) line up on the surface of the HA granules, adjacent to some previously mineralised bone. The section displays undisturbed vascularisation and intensive bone regeneration, obviously influenced by the HA particles. Many blood vessels are present (*b*). (Test 91 right, Collapat E, 3 weeks) MG, × 150

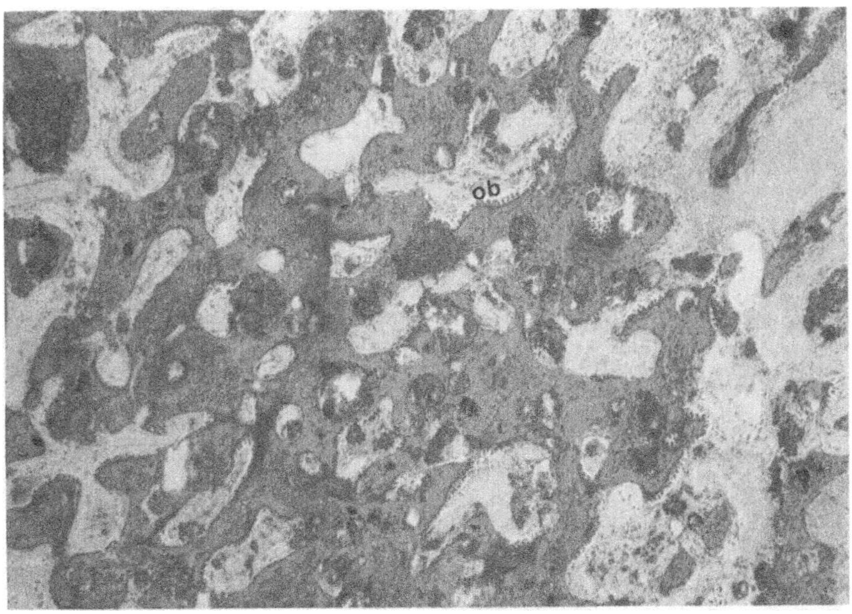

Fig. 5.70. The HA granules (*dark grey*) are already completely surrounded by regenerated bone, massive numbers of osteoblasts (*ob*), and many blood vessels. The implant has not interfered with vascularisation of the defect cavity in any way. (Test 91 right, Collapat E, 3 weeks) MG, × 90

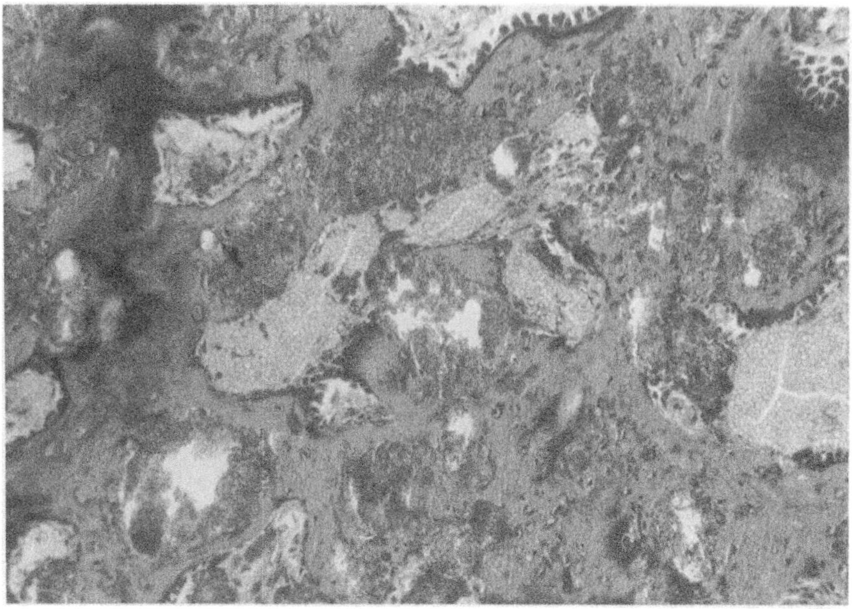

Fig. 5.71. Enlarged sector from Fig. 5.70, × 210

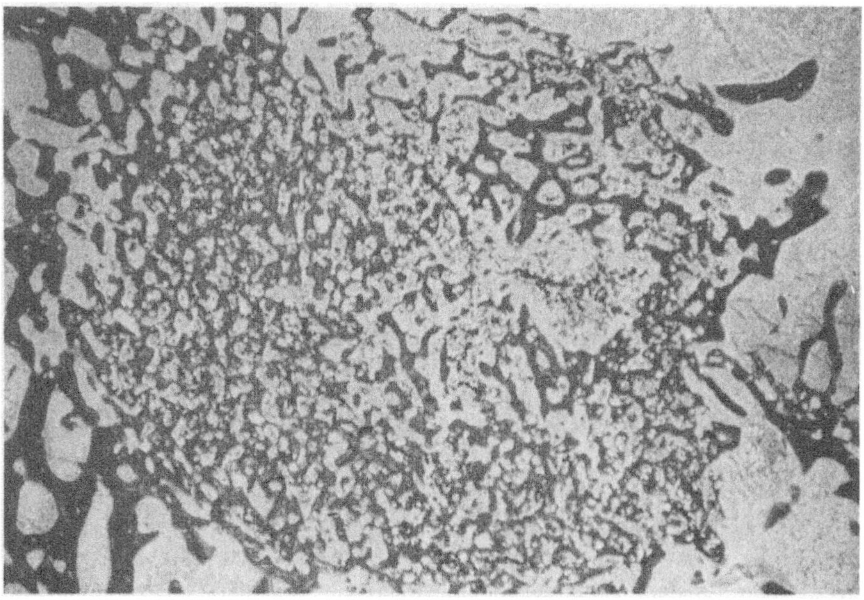

Fig. 5.72. Complete bony re-structuring of the defect cavity, with the exception of a small remaining defect. (Test 68 right, Collapat E, 4 weeks) MG, × 15

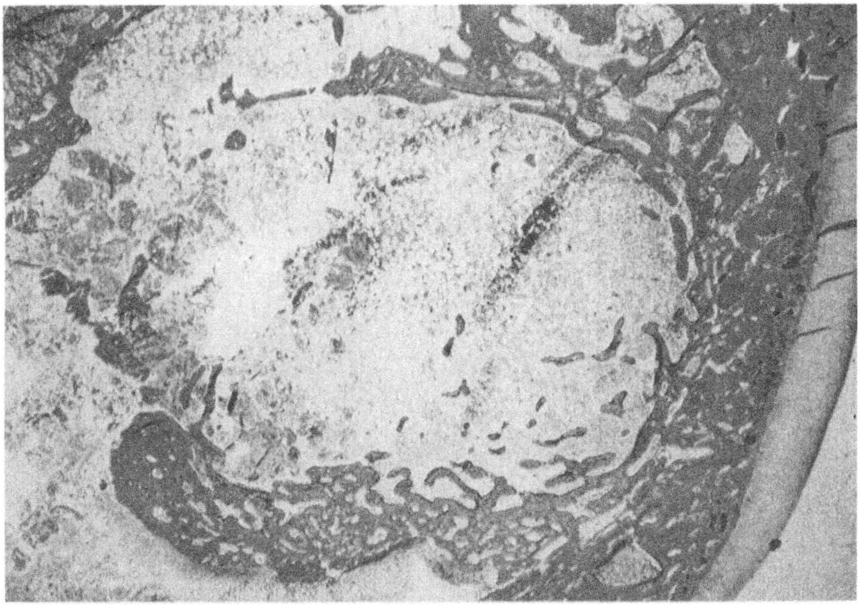

Fig. 5.73. The empty cavity on the opposite side exhibits only slight peripheral bone regeneration; note the difference between the two sides, compare with Fig. 5.72 (Test 68 left, empty cavity, 4 weeks) MG, × 15

This observation is of particular importance because so far it has been taken for granted that osteoconduction always proceeds via the detour of an osteoclastic resorption of a given, e. g. transplanted bone tissue. Since this osteoclastic form of osteoconduction is well documented, our test results suggest the existence of a *completely different, distinct form of osteoconduction*. We will revert to this concept in more detail in the concluding discussion.

The tight-meshed bony reconstruction of the defect cavity recurred *in all preparations* up to 6 weeks. In the gaps in the meshwork, *normal bone-marrow tissue* had formed. Inflammatory defensive reactions were not observed. In one section after 8 weeks, there was a central gap where no bone had formed, but which also contained no apatite granules. This result is particularly impressive because it demonstrates that bone regeneration *occurs in areas where an apatite implant is present, and is absent in implant-free areas*. Obviously, this defect cavity had not been completely filled with implantation material.

Subsequent developments involved *remodelling* of the regenerated bone. The bone became wider, and appeared more mature, but tended to decrease in quantity. It appeared that *excess bone with regard to biomechanical requirements,* which had been formed during the initial massive osteostimulation, was now undergoing secondary resorption. It was also obvious that the apatite granules did not interfere with bone remodelling in any way. The granules appeared to be tolerated and integrated by the bone es though they were equivalent to it (Fig. 5.74).

The ceramised apatite particles were still recognizable as such even *after 8 months;* they were resorbed very slowly, and retained their close bond with the bone (Fig. 5.75).

Quantitative comparison of the 2- through 12-week sections of the first Collapat E series with empty cavities gave in the Collapat E series a minimum of 13.8%, a maximum of 59.4% and an average value of 38.4% (Table 5.15). On the other hand, the relative surface areas of regenerated bone in the empty cavities varied between 1.6% and 16.7%, and averaged 8.5%. If one compares these averages, in cavities with Collapat E, *4.5 times as much bone as in empty cavities* was formed (Figs. 5.76 and 5.77).

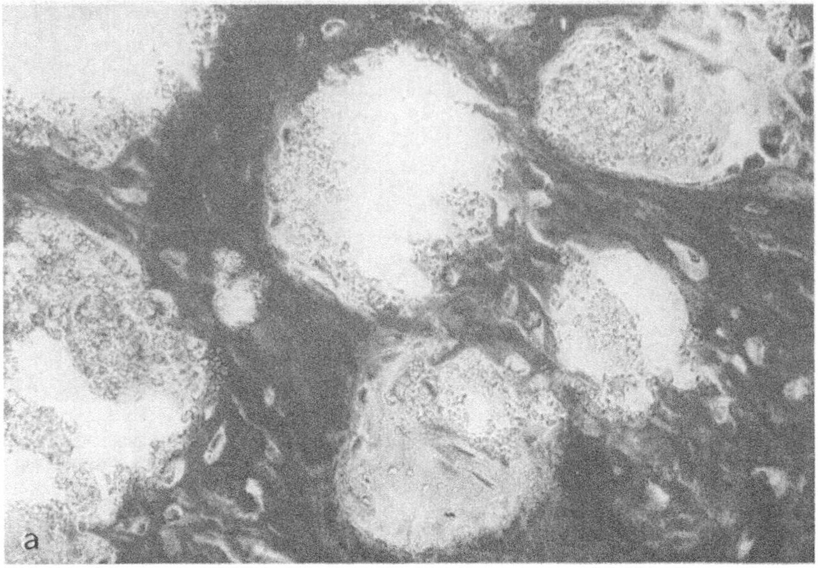

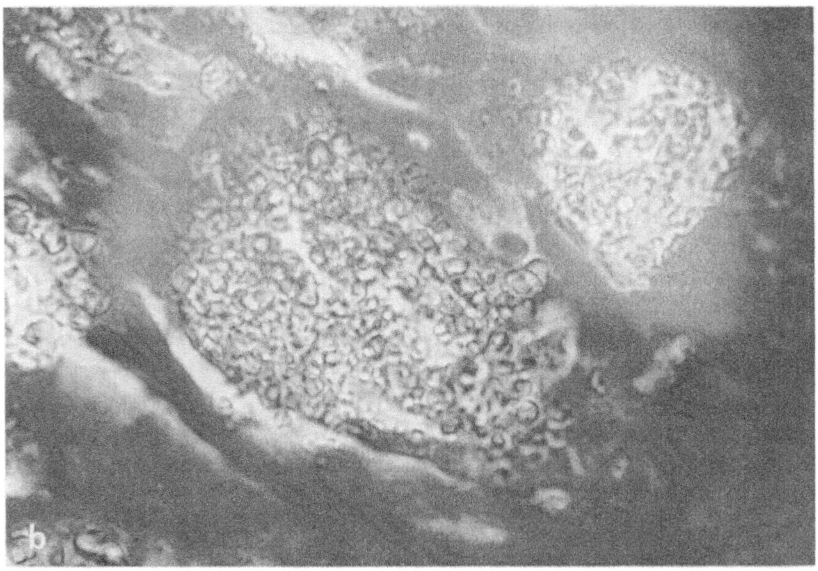

Fig. 5.74a, b. The hydroxyapatite granules are completely embedded in regenerated bone. There is no separating layer of connective tissue. Osteocytes can be detected on the surface of the granules. The HA particles have been integrated into the bone as though they were "equivalent" to it. (Test 67 left, Collapat E, 4 weeks) MG, **a** × 150. **b** × 300

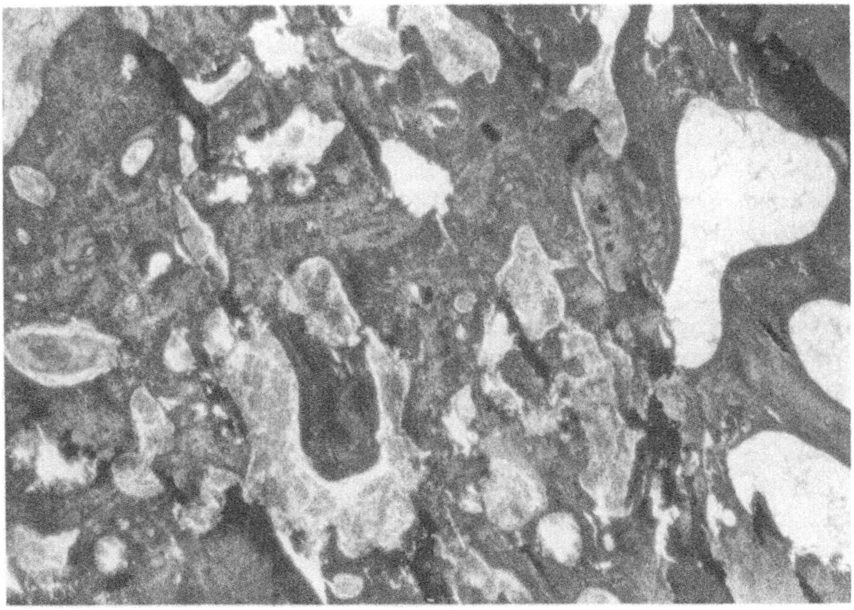

Fig. 5.75. The strong bond between apatite and regenerated bone persists for a long time. Bone remodelling is not disturbed by the small HA particles; they are resorbed very slowly and obviously retain their "bone affinity". (Test 78 right, Collapat E, 8 months) MG, × 50

Table 5.15. Surface-area measurements of regenerated bone 2 weeks–8 months after Collapat E implantation

Test number	Duration	Bone regeneration measured per unit surface area (%)
69L	2 weeks	13.8
71R	2 weeks	21.9
91R	3 weeks	44.7
92R	3 weeks	66.3
93R	3 weeks	43.9
94R	3 weeks	40.5
95R	3 weeks	40.5
67L	4 weeks	51.1
68R	4 weeks	42.6
87R	4 weeks	39.8
88R	4 weeks	17.4
89R	4 weeks	43.4
90R	4 weeks	59.6
74R	6 weeks	59.4
75L	6 weeks	51.6
70R	8 weeks	38.2
72R	8 weeks	25.6
73R	12 weeks	46.8
76L	12 weeks	37.7
78R	8 months	33.2

The experimental results were verified for statistical significance in the Mann-Whitney U-test. This test demonstrated with an error probability of $P < 0.002$ – i. e. beyond any doubt – that the collagen-apatite mixed preparation (Collapat E) has a promoting effect on bone regeneration, when compared with empty control cavities.

Tests comparing Collapat E as a bone-replacement material with autogenic spongiosa over 3–4 weeks gave the following results: for Collapat E, a minimum of 17.4%, a maximum of 66.3% and an average of 44%; for autogenous spongiosa, a minimum of 23.3%, a maximum of 52.3% and an average value of 32.4%. Although the results obtained with Collapat E implants were better than those with autogenic spongiosa, a significant difference in a statistical test could not be shown, since the standard deviation of the test results was too large, and the number of tests was still too limited. It is particularly noteworthy that with the best bone-transplantation material, autogenic spongiosa, no better results were obtained in beds with high regenerative capacity than with the bone-replacement material Collapat E (Figs. 5.78 and 5.79).

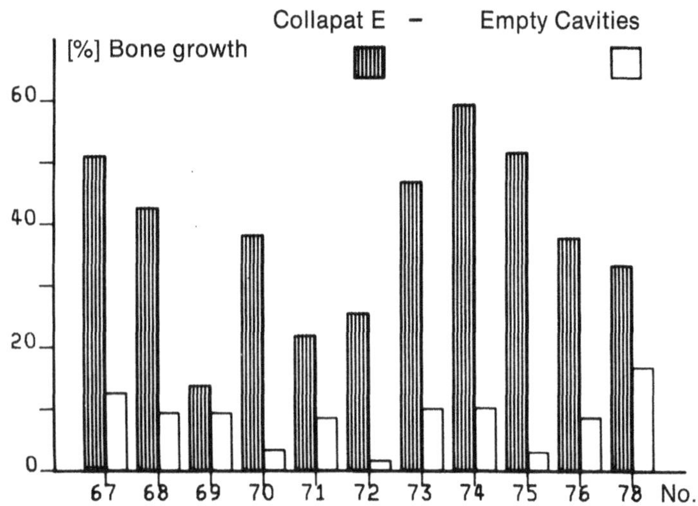

Fig. 5.76. Bone regeneration with Collapat E compared to regeneration in empty cavities. The difference in favour of Collapat E is highly significant

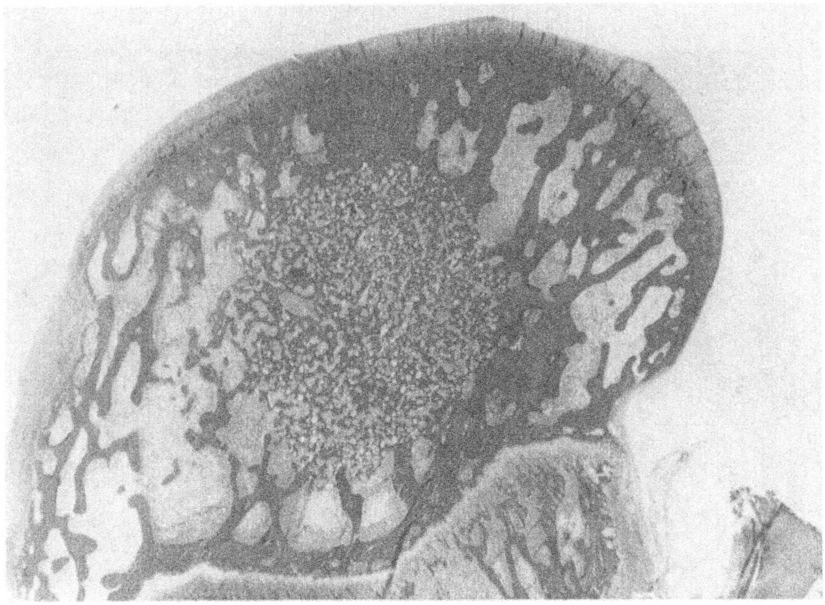

Fig. 5.77. The defect is completely filled with bone after 6 weeks with Collapat E. (Test 74)

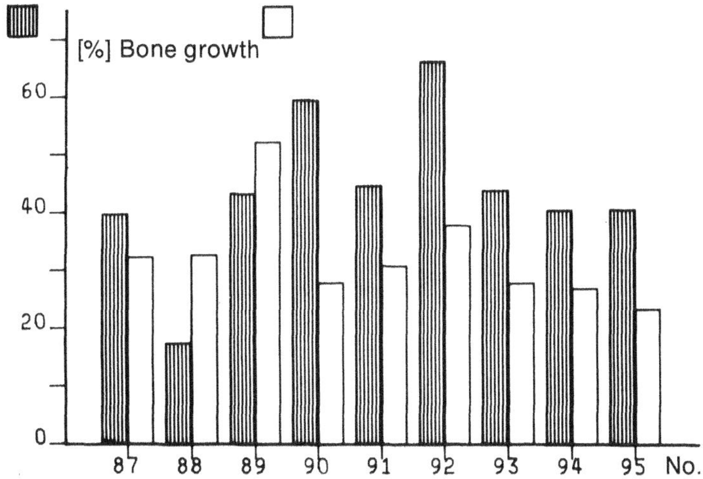

Fig. 5.78. Results of bone regeneration with Collapat E in comparison with autogenic spongiosa transplantation. The average value for autogenic spongiosa ($x = 32.4$; standard deviation $s = 8.5$) is lower than for Collapat E ($x = 44.0$; $s = 13.7$). However, a statistically significant difference could not be demonstrated in this test series

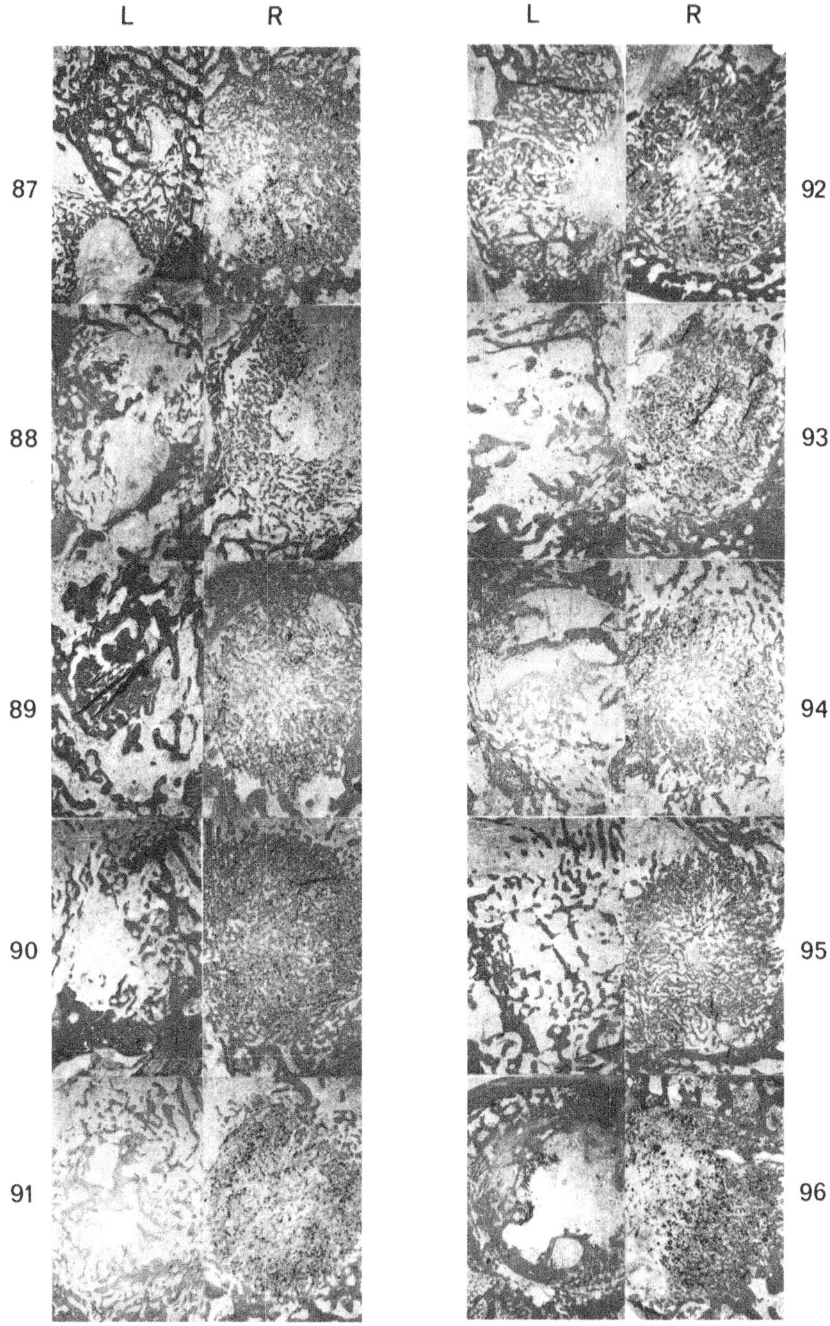

Fig. 5.79. Series of survey photographs. Almost all preparations with Collapat E show complete regeneration of the defect; *L*, autogenic spongiosa; *R*, Collapat E (3 and 4 weeks, test number *next to the photograph*) MG, × 4

5.4.2.10 Totally Deproteinated Natural Mineral Bone (Pyrost)

Twelve experiments were made using Pyrost as an implant. Histological evaluation after *2 weeks* showed practically uninhibited vascularisation of the bone defect. Obviously, the implant did not interfere with this process in any manner. At this stage, a *large quantity of regenerated bone* was already detectable on the surfaces of the Pyrost implant, with bone regeneration again occurring in direct contact with the implantation material. In this respect, the histological findings resembled those obtained using the fine-particle dispersion of apatite granules. Due to the structure of Pyrost, with fine elongated bars, *widespread formation of bone trabeculae* in the marrow cavities of the implant was observed from the outset, and developed, at the earliest stage, into an apparently *natural* network of regenerated bone. Many osteoblasts were present, but there was *no evidence of a defensive reaction* against the implant. Bone regeneration was accompanied everywhere by fine vascularisation (Figs. 5.80–5.86).

As in the case of ceramised apatite particles, some of the implant crumbled away during the histological cutting process, but again remained partly intact where it was in contact with regenerated bone. Here as well, the existence of a *strong physico-chemical bond between the implant surface and the regenerated bone* was suggested.

As with the collagen-apatite mixed preparations, there was intensive bone regeneration with Pyrost up to the 4th week (Fig. 5.87).

With this implantation material, it is also remarkable that bone regeneration sometimes occurred directly on the surface of the implant. Furthermore, dense callous formed in between the mesh of the implant. The implant was firmly incorporated and integrated in regenerated bone. After *4 weeks,* the defect cavity was almost completely restructured with regenerated bone.

In the subsequent course of the experiment, bone remodelling again became the principal process. The bone trabeculae became broader and seemed more mature. Also, after *6 weeks, normal bone marrow* had regenerated in the interstices. When the implant had not been placed absolutely correctly, bone regeneration was regularly observed on the surface of the implant material in the region of the femoral canal, as in epiphyseal implantation (Figs. 5.88–5.90).

The conspicuous granulomatous defensive and connective-tissue reactions seen with Kiel splinters did not occur with Pyrost implants. The implanted material was only resorbed very slowly, and was still present almost in its entirety *after 8 months;* the strong

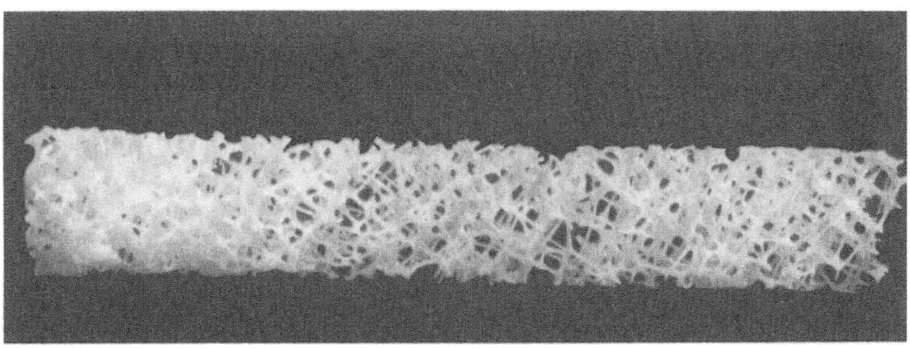

Fig. 5.80. Macroscopic view of the Pyrost implant, showing filigree structure with large gaps

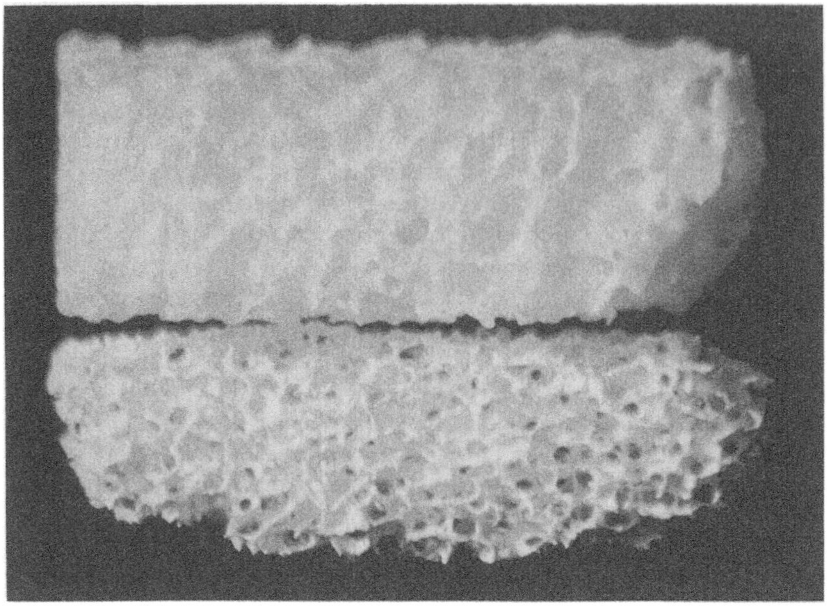

Fig. 5.81. Two adjacent pieces of spongy bone treated according to the Kiel procedure (*above*) and after Pyrost preparation (*below*). Considerably larger pores are seen in the "transparent" Pyrost in comparison to the Kiel bone splinter, in which the mineral structure is still obscured by the collagen structure

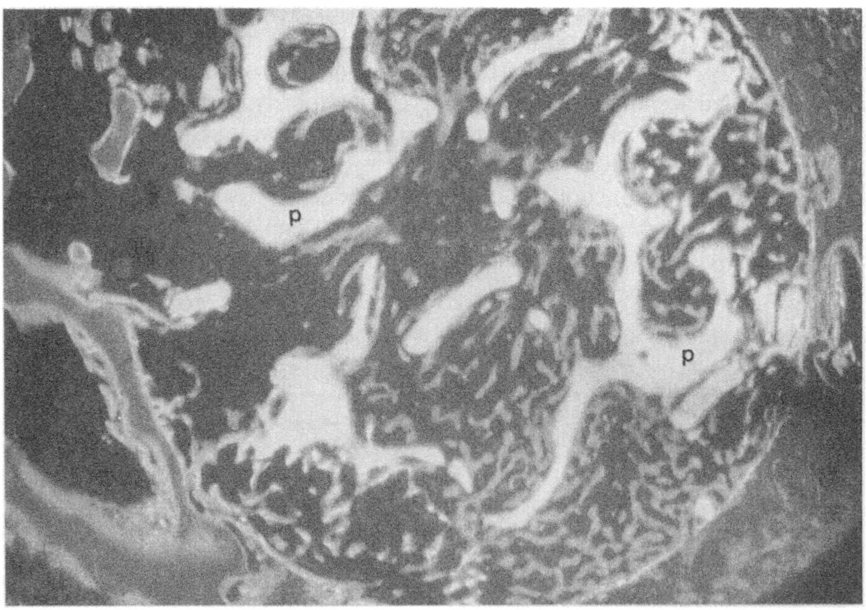

Fig. 5.82. Fluorescence micrograph of early bone regeneration on Pyrost. The brightly shining Pyrost implant (p) is surrounded everywhere, right to the centre, by regenerated bone. (Test 20 left, Pyrost, 2 weeks) × 15

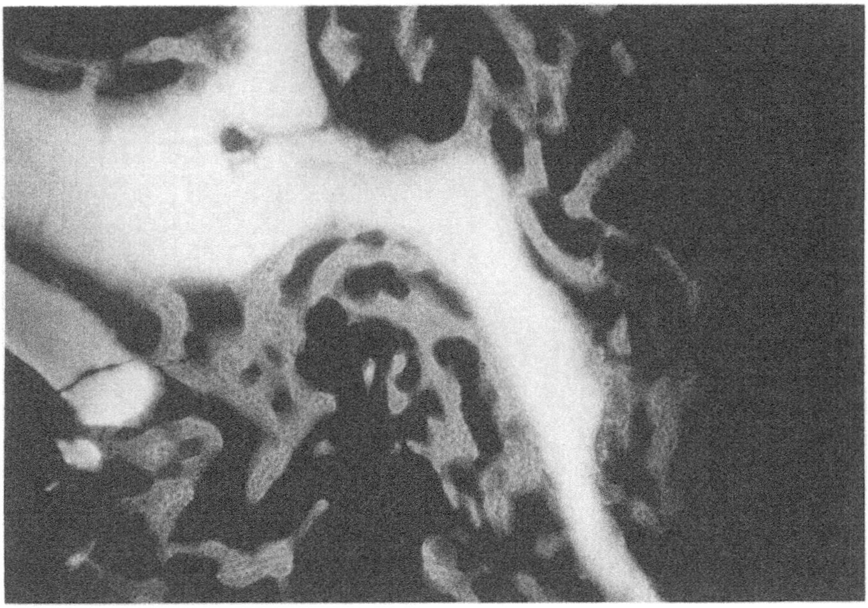

Fig. 5.83. Enlarged sector from Fig. 5.82. × 50

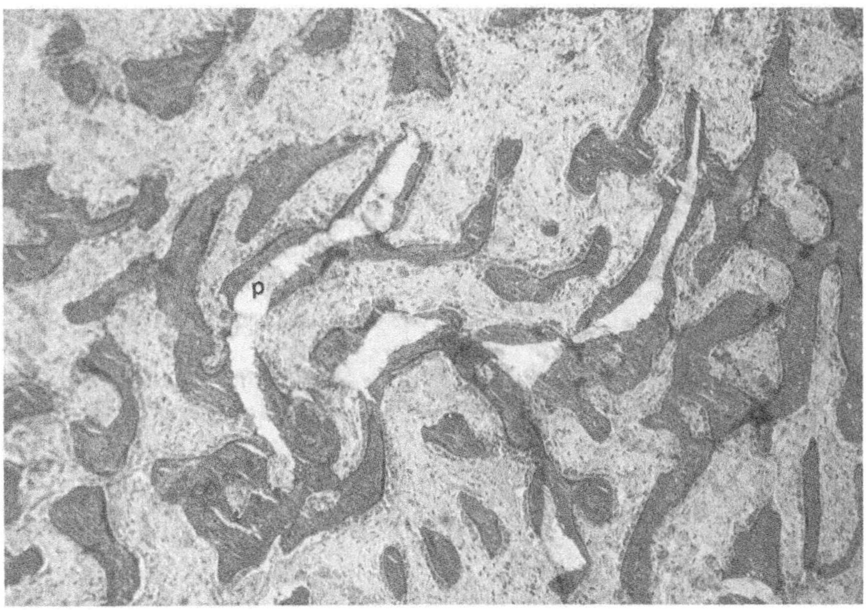

Fig. 5.84. Vigorous bone regeneration on the surface of the Pyrost implant (*p*), which has partially crumbled away during the cutting process. As with synthetic HA ceramic material, there is no connective tissue layer between implant and bone. (Test 20, left, Pyrost, 2 weeks) MG, × 40

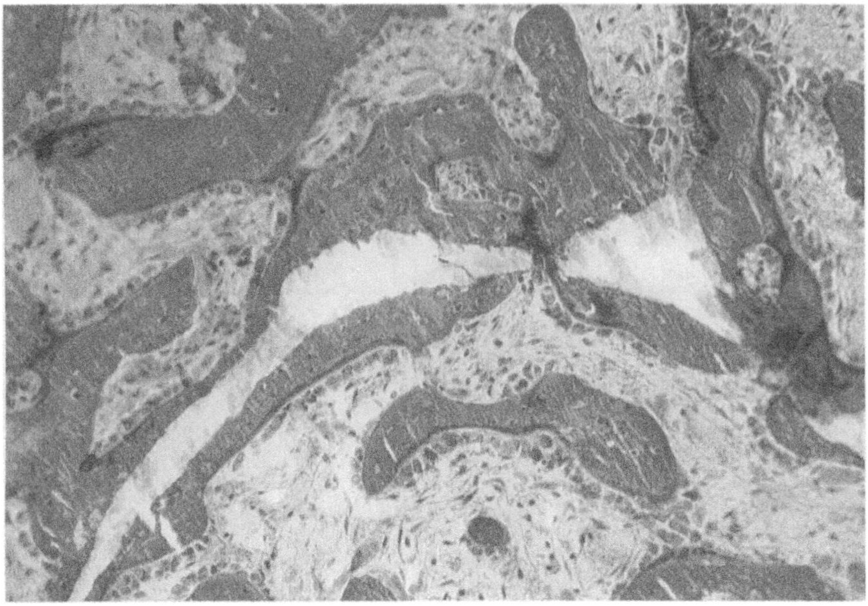

Fig. 5.85. Enlarged sector from Fig. 5.84. × 100

bond between the implanted material and the regenerated bone continued to exist. There was no evidence that the implant interfered with bone remodelling. Pyrost also appeared to be accepted as "equivalent" tissue and incorporated into the bone. The resulting network of regenerated bone surrounding the implant and filling the interstices was as dense as, and sometimes even denser than the surrounding intact bone structures. Therefore, *the regenerated bone is also capable of standing up to physiological and mechanical loads* (Fig. 5.91).

To summarise, it can be concluded that sintered natural mineral bone (Pyrost) also obviously exerts an *intense stimulus on osteoregeneration.* The stimulus, however, only becomes fully effective when there is unhindered vascularisation and in the absence of defensive reactions. As in the case of Kiel-splinter implants, the colour contrast between implanted Pyrost and regenerated bone was not strong enough for automated histomorphometry. Some of the Pyrost crumbled away when the sections were cut, sometimes carrying regenerated bone with it, so that while the histological sections were of sufficient quality for qualitative assessment, they did not permit histomorphometric evaluation of this test series. Accurate histomorphometric evaluation of Pyrost implants will be the subject of a further project.

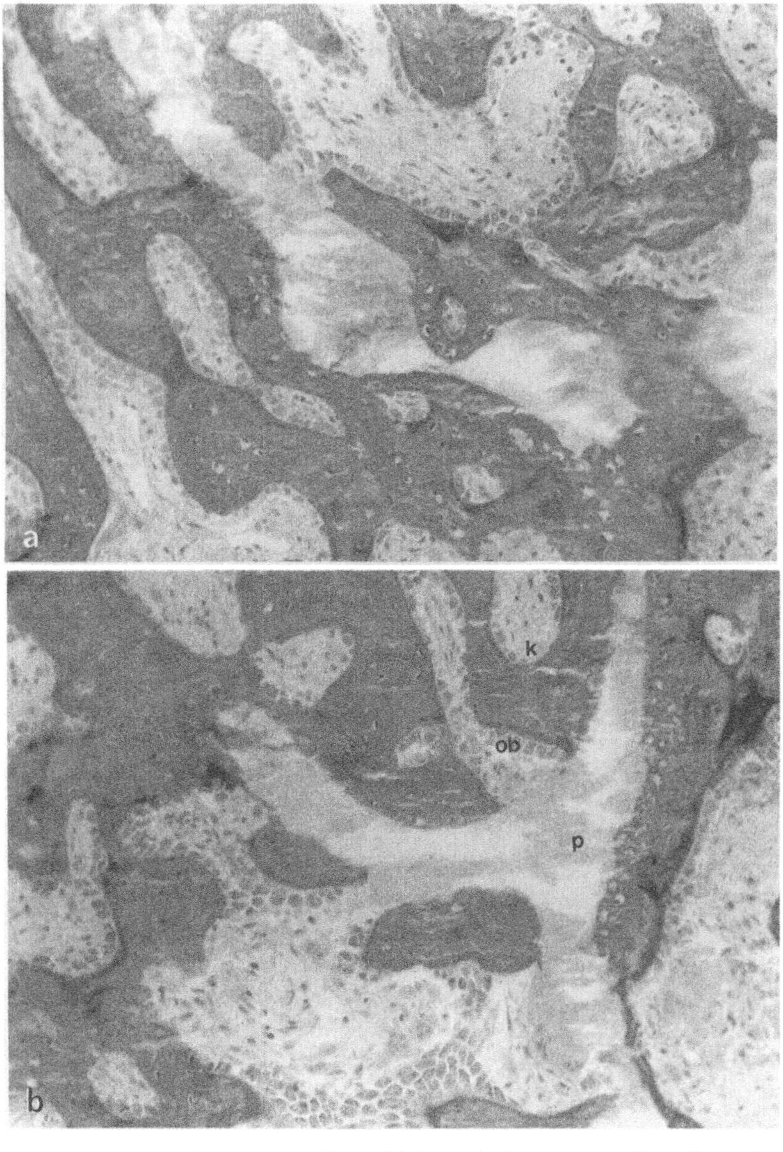

Fig. 5.86 a, b. Pyrost (p) surrounded by regenerated bone (k). Intensive bone regeneration with massive numbers of osteoblasts (ob) can be seen. There is also no separating layer of connective tissue between the bone and the Pyrost. There is absolutely no defensive reaction against the implant. (Test 24 left) MG, × 100

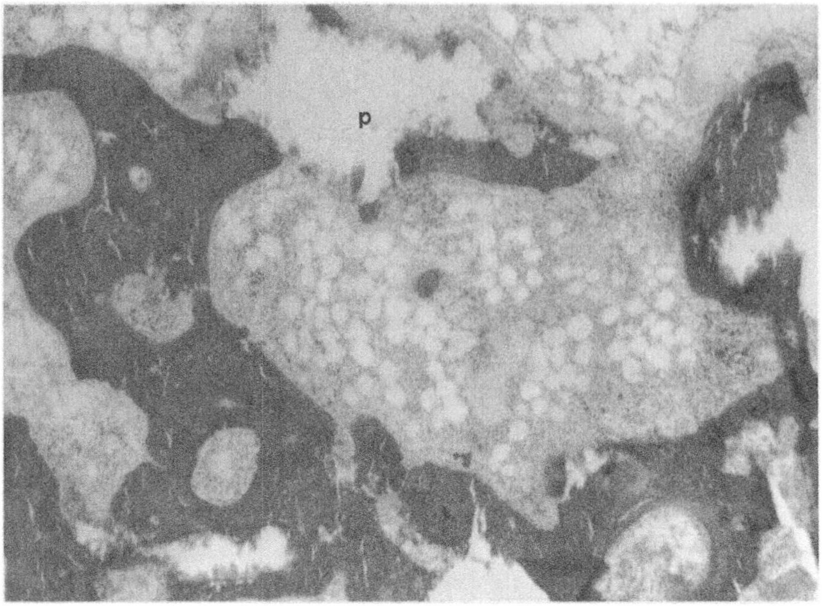

Fig. 5.87. In contrast to the "Kiel bone splinters", the immunogen-free implantation material Pyrost (*p*) is surrounded by large amounts of regenerated bone; adjacent to it is inconspicuous regenerated marrow tisse. (Test 18 left, 4 weeks) MG, × 100

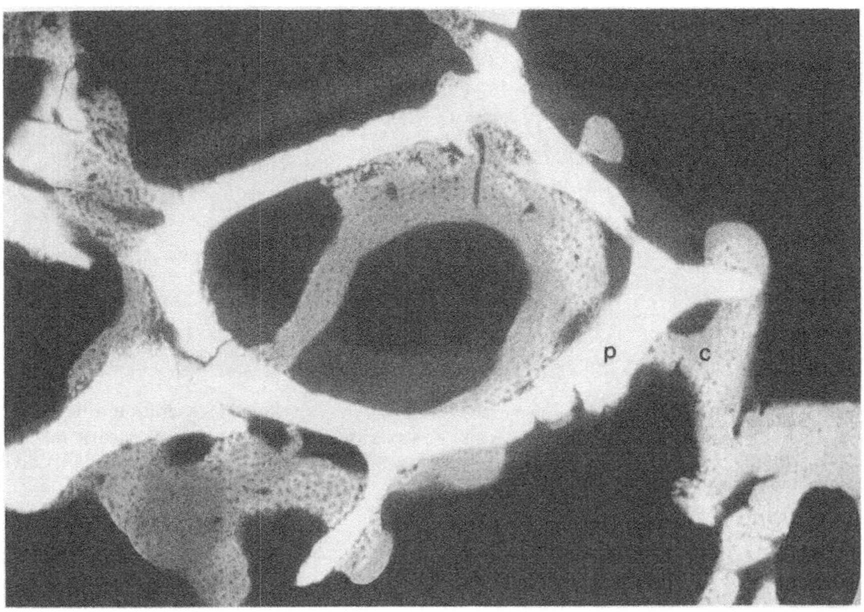

Fig. 5.88. The small Pyrost bars (*p*) appear bright white with high contrast due to sintering. On their inner and outer surfaces, abundant regenerated bone tissue is visible (*c*). (Test 13 left, 8 weeks, microradiograph) × 60

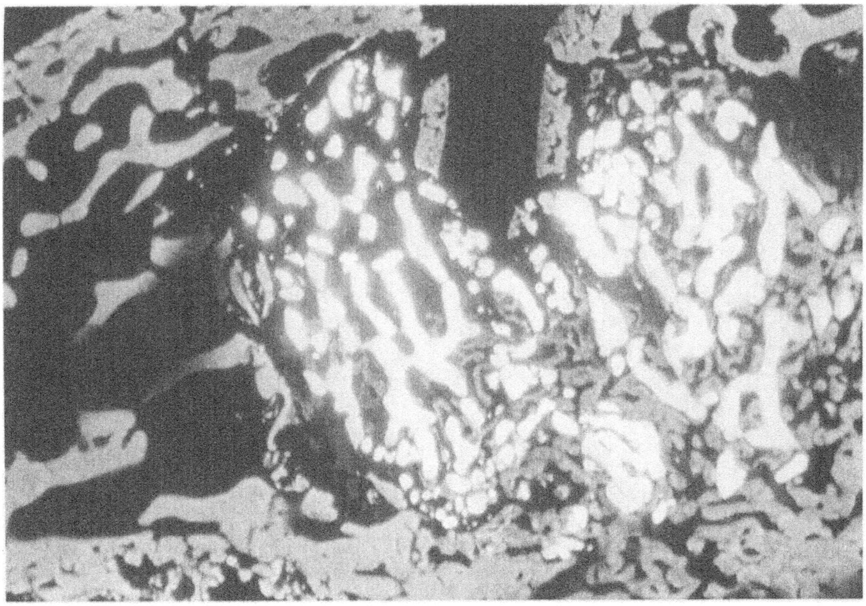

Fig. 5.89. Pyrost (*white*) is completely surrounded with regenerated bone. *Black areas* correspond to marrow tissue and blood vessels. (Test 23 left, 4 weeks, microradiograph) × 15

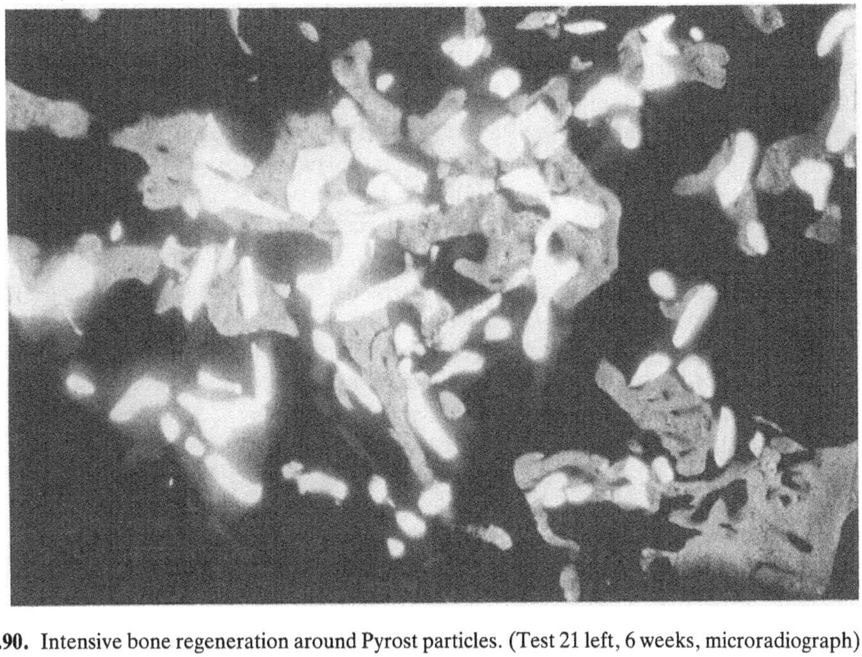

Fig. 5.90. Intensive bone regeneration around Pyrost particles. (Test 21 left, 6 weeks, microradiograph) × 20

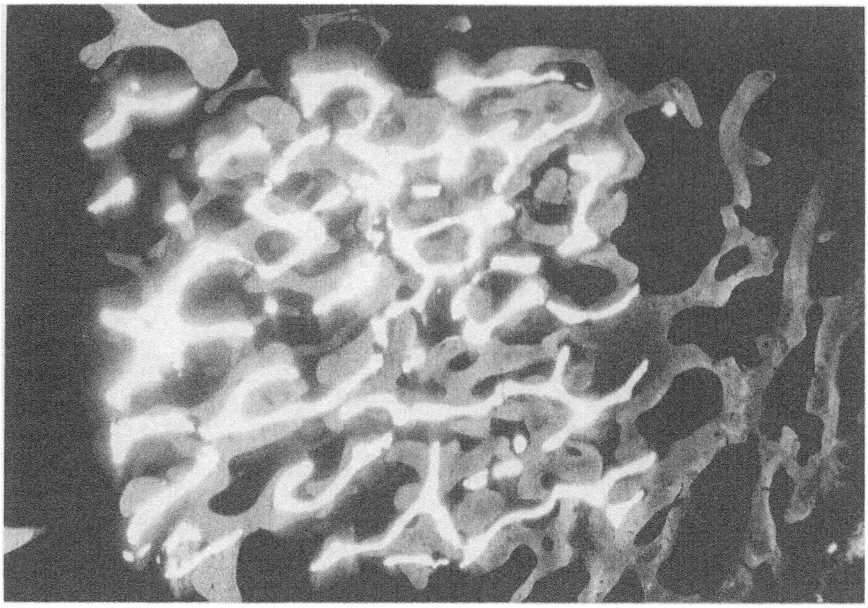

Fig. 5.91. Long-term test with Pyrost, 8 months. The *bright* Pyrost implant is still almost totally preserved. The entire bone-defect area is filled with regenerated bone. Pyrost and regenerated bone are closely linked together. (Test 15 left, microradiograph) × 15

5.4.2.11 Synthetic Porous Apatite Ceramic Materials

For comparison purposes, we performed two pilot experiments that tested the commercial preparation Ceros 80 (from Synthes; Synthes Bulletin 1983), which is offered commercially for filling bone defects either instead of or in combination with autogenic spongiosa. This preparation is also made up of a hydroxyapatite ceramic material and, according to information from the manufacturer, has a pore size of 200–400 μm. This material is also available commercially in the form of several more or less porous, pressure-resistant articles for use, e. g. for intercorporal spondylodesis and total replacement of vertebrae (Fig. 5.92).

In our pilot experiments with this material, we found intensive *osteoregeneration on the implant surface* after *4 weeks,* including the superficial pores (Figs. 5.93 and 5.94). In contrast to the collagen-apatite mixed preparations and the Pyrost implants, which have much larger pores, osteogenesis occurred only in the superficial pores; the *central pores remained completely bone-free.* It was obvious that the pore size was insufficient, and the implant inhibited vascularisation of the defect, as was found by Schweiberer (1970) for Kiel bone splinters, so that it was itself exposed to mechanical loads on a permanent basis. In view of its *inadequate long-term resistance to fatigue,* this implant is at risk of fatigue fracture, since in spite of bony incorporation the bone cannot grow through the implant because of impaired vascularisation. The role of a bone-replacement material should not be that of a permanent bone replacement, but rather the stimulation of autogenous bone regeneration, as has been explained earlier. Although the Ceros 80 implant had the same chemical composition as the apatite in the collagen-apatite mixed preparation, it must be considered an inferior bone-replacement material because of its unfavourable application form with insufficiently small interstices between the meshes.

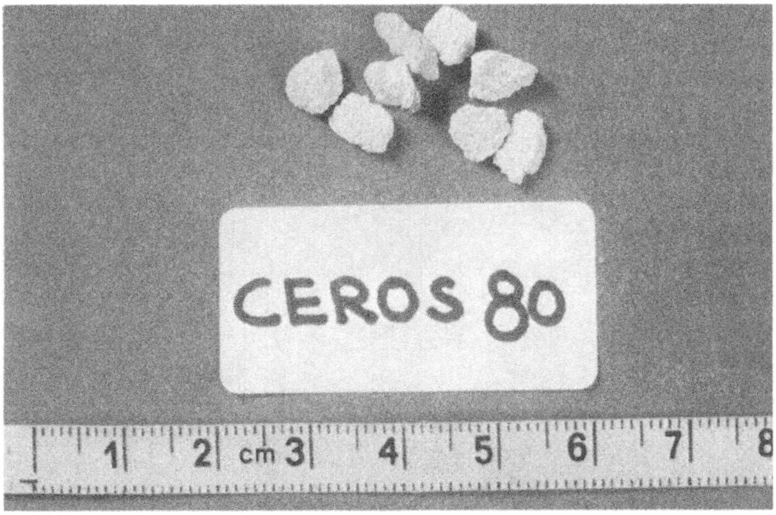

Fig. 5.92. Ceros 80 (Synthes), porous hydroxyapatite ceramic material in particle form

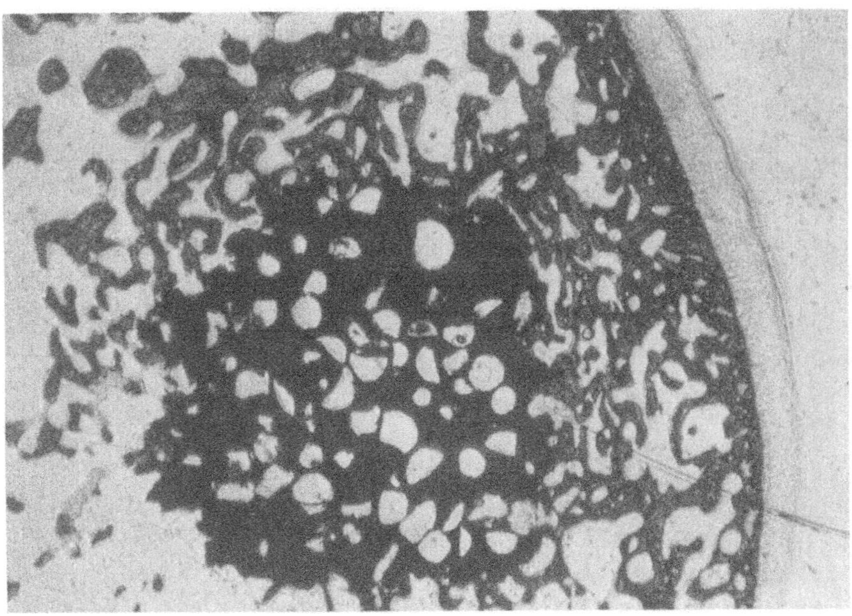

Fig. 5.93. Bone regenerates on the implant surface, but not in the deeper pores. With Collapat E, the defect had been filled completely with regenerated bone by this time; *black,* Ceros with pores; *grey,* bone. (Test 84, Ceros 80, 4 weeks) MG, × 15

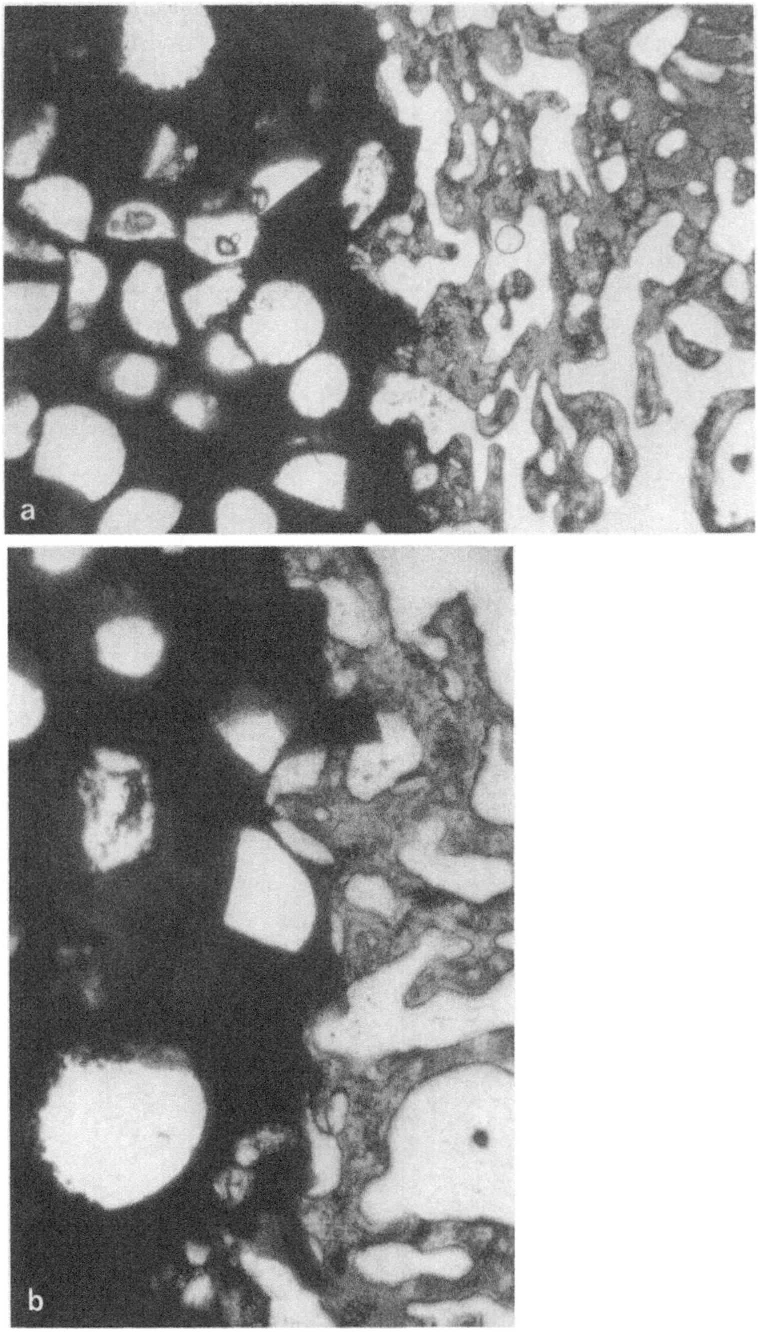

Fig. 5.94 a, b. The implant promotes good bone regeneration on the surface, but impairs bone growth within the defect cavity, in a barrier-like manner, because of its excessive bulk and overly small pores. (Test 84, Ceros 80, 4 weeks) **a** × 40. **b** Another sector, MG, × 100

6 Discussion of the Experimental Results

The assessment of bone-replacement materials is only possible against the background of current experience with bone transplants. It is generally accepted that autogenous spongiosa and bone marrow are the only bone-transplants with an osteogenic effect, i.e. only these grafts contain cells which are capable of permanent proliferation and osteoregeneration.

At first, before the onset of immunological defensive reactions, allogenic spongiosa is also capable of inducing osteoblastic proliferation; this, however, is stopped by immunological defensive processes after 8–9 days and is suppressed more or less completely according to the strength of the immunological response. Further bone regeneration under the influence of such transplants proceeds indirectly via creeping substitution [W. Axhausen 1952; Schweiberer et al. 1981]. The immunological reaction against cortical allografts in slighter due to the lower content of immunogenic cells. However, cortical allografts are very slowly revascularised and often remain necrotic. Nevertheless allografts play an increasing role in tumour surgery, revision hip asthroplasty and joint reconstruction.

In xenogenic bone transplants, the defensive reactions are so violent that they also interfere with the body's own bone regeneration for a prolonged period. They must therefore be regarded as unsuitable transplant materials. This also applies, though to a lesser degree, to partially deproteinated Kiel bone splinters. Our experiments have shown that Kiel splinters also induce a strong, although not immediate, defensive reaction which leads to resorption of the bone splinters themselves and impedes the body's own bone-regeneration mechanisms.

The bone-replacement materials investigated in the course of this project are of course not capable of osteogenic bone regeneration originating from the implant, since they do not contain bone-forming cells. In this respect autogenic spongiosa continues to be clearly superior to all other implant or transplant materials. Therefore, it will still be necessary to use autogenous bone or marrows in future when the conditions for healing of the bone defect are unfavourable due to the poor regenerative capacity of the recipient bed (inadequate circulation, infection, very large bone-substance defects and local deficiency of osteogenic cells).

In the discussion of our experimental results we must first turn our attention to the test model. In all animal experiments the question as to whether the test results are applicable to man needs to be answered. However, with regard to osteoregeneration in particular, past experience has shown that previous tests on laboratory animals have correctly assessed the potential of and predicted the problems of different, i.e. autogenic, allogenic and xenogenic bone-transplant materials. Only animal experiments have made it possible to recognise the complex problems, advantages and disadvantages of different bone transplants. Results obtained with bone grafts in animal experiments are generally accepted today as being valid for man. This has been confirmed by clinical experience with various transplant materials. Animal experiments are therefore undoubtedly of great importance in the study of bone regeneration. This applies equally to the different bone-replacement materials.

Eitel et al. (1981) studied the applicability of animal-experiment results to the regeneration of human long bone and concluded that the usual methods of osteological research provide an acceptable morphological picture of the osteogenic repair process and that the results obtained are transferable to man provided that the skeletal age and the physiological load parameters are comparable. A certain limitation which needs to be considered rests in the fact that Eitel et al. performed all their studies on dogs; whether these results also apply to experiments with rabbits therefore remains an open issue.

Bone-regeneration studies on metaphyseal bone defects, particularly in the rabbit, are always criticised because the healing conditions in this model are said to be so favourable that osteoregeneration would be possible even with the worst implant material. For this reason we included a large series of control experiments in this project. These control experiments demonstrated that spontaneous osteoregeneration obviously has its limits even in rabbit spongy beds. No significant bone regeneration was obtained with some implant materials (gelatin, Kiel splinters and bone matrix).

The test model used in this project, which was renommended by Mittelmeier, and previously used successfully by Nizard (1981), with 6 mm bore holes in the rabbit femoral condyle, is definitely not capable of spontaneous bone regeneration. In fact, the defect remains visible after weeks and even months. It is only partly compensated by bony reinforcement of the peripheral structures around the defect. Bony reconstruction of the defect itself does not occur. Schenk and Willenegger (1977) also demonstrated with defects drilled in the rabbit cortex that primary bone regeneration has its limits, and does not occur in larger drilled defect cavities.

Our explanation for this phenomenon is that the size of the bone defect in relation to its surrounding bone plays a decisive role here. It is probable that, beyond a certain defect size, the bone-regeneration process is disturbed to such an extent that spontaneous regeneration is no longer possible. Our control experiments show that the experimental model we have used is valid for the morphometric investigation of bone regeneration in beds of high regenerative capacity.

The histomorphometric technique used in our experiments requires separate discussion. There are several possibilities for error in this technique (in recognition and interactive marking of the bone defect on the screen, staining of the bone preparations, selection of the slides from the section series, the number of evaluated sections and in some cases the small number of tests). However, it should be borne in mind that these error possibilities apply equally to the tested bone-replacement materials, to autogenic spongiosa and to empty cavities. The actual test results show such large differences between the various preparations that these differences remain obvious even after allowing for a certain margin of error. Also, in order to minimise the error margin, multiple measurements were performed. Generally three, and in one test series (Collapat E against empty cavities) even ten, different bone sections per test were evaluated. The differences between the results obtained with the tested bone-replacement material and with empty cavities were so large that for each individual test a stastistically significant difference in favour of Collapat E could be shown. Considering the very large variations in results from test series to test series, the error margin associated with the measuring technique seems to be limited and the test results thus sufficiently reliable.

We pointed out earlier that autogenic spongiosa is clearly superior and will always be superior to all other transplant and implant materials on the basis of its osteogenic potency. The question then arises whether it would not be the best approach to use this optimal material for all indications. As explained in the discussion of autogenic spongiosa in Sect. 3.2, we do not favour this procedure because transplantation of autogenic spongiosa also has disadvantages associated with bone remoral, which are often underestimated and which we will not discuss here yet again. The indiscriminate use of autogenic spongiosa to fill all bone defects is not the correct approach. Differentiated criteria of indication are required, according to the healing conditions prevailing. The patient should not be burdened with the draw-backs associated with autogenic bone transplants when the goal – bone healing – can be achieved in a simpler way.

One alternative is allogenic bone transplantation, although this always proceeds indirectly and only after a considerable delay, via creeping substitution. Apart from the immunological problems associated with allogenic bone transplantation, in the past not enough attention has been given to the problem of local or parenteral transmission of infectious and systemic diseases. The procedure for allogenic bone transplantation described by Knöfler (1978) is no longer acceptable today and involves excessive risk for the patient. Either these risks must be eliminated by exercising extreme care in the management of the bone bank, with regard to donor selection and testing of the transplants, which requires considerable resources, or other alternatives must be considered. Because of the considerable expense and the remaining risks and problems associated with allogenic bone transplants today, this technique is also limited to certain indications (joint reconstruction, very big bone defects).

For this reason a world-wide search for suitable bone-replacement materials is in progress. This search is proceeding in three independent directions, which will again be compared with each other and have been grouped under the key-words "collagen", "bone matrix" and "calcium phosphate".

The objective we set ourselves in this project was a quantitative comparison of the osteoregenerative potential of various bone-replacement materials. Both collagen alone and bone matrix showed partially favourable bone regeneration in one or the other experiment, consistent with favourable reports from other authors, but the promoting effect on osteoregeneration was not shown to be statistically significant in our test series. Although bone matrix (BMP) has been proven by numerous authors to be osteoinductive, this material is not yet available for clinical practice. The extraction of pure "osteogenin" remains to be seen.

Hydroxyapatite ceramic material in the form presented here proved to be far superior to all other bone-replacement materials tested. This could be shown primarily by quantitative comparison of the collagen-apatite mixed preparation Collapat E with empty cavities and also in comparison to autogenic spongiosa. The promoting effect on bone regeneration seen with the pyrolised, sintered, natural mineral bone Pyrost was also impressive.

It is, however, by no means irrelevant which application form is chosen for implantation of the hydroxyapatite ceramic into the body. In this context we wish to emphasize Schweiberer's statement (1970) that osteoregeneration can only proceed if vascularisation of the defect is possible. The stimulation of bone regeneration by the hydroxyapatite implant must, therefore, not interfere with the vascularisation of the defect if it is to be effective. For this reason, the relatively compact apatite ceramic materials, with small pores are not very suitable. Because of its insufficient long-term fatigue strength, implantation of this material would be risky for some indications despite the good bony incorporation. A porous, more or less compact apatite ceramic material is probably bound to fail as a permanent replacement, e.g. of a vertebra. Shima et al. (1979) observed compression of the implant with ventral or dorsal dislocation in 70% of the cases of cervical spondylodesis in their animal experiments, and we have to warn here against the use of this material as a replacement for a vertebra.

While originating from the same materials, the fine particle dispersion in the collagen-apatite mixed preparation suggested by Mittelmeier (personal communication), on the one hand, and the wide-meshed filigree structure of the Pyrost implant, on the other hand, are basically different from all other application forms. The Mittelmeier's theory that the osteoregenerative potential of materials in this form would become fully effective through multi-centric bone regeneration around the dispersed hydroxyapatite particles or the widemeshed Pyrost spongiosa was clearly confirmed by our results. With this application form, the vascularisation of the defect required for effective osteoregeneration is not impaired and the promotion of osteoregeneration can become fully effective when cells capable of bone formation are brought into contact with the implant by the blood vessels. The excellent biocompatibility of the material, which has been reported by all researchers working with hydroxyapatite as an implantation material, is also confirmed by our own investigations.

In addition, our own experiments reveal new information about bone regeneration under the influence of inorganic compounds. The conclusion arrived at by Schweiberer (1970) that inorganic compounds do not play a role in osteogenesis is demonstrably incorrect on the basis of our results. Also, Urist et al. (1984) found a 12-times-higher rate of bone regeneration when bone matrix (BMP) was mixed with beta-tricalcium phosphate. The mechanism of action is not yet clear, although it is probably the same effect as occurred in our own studies with hydroxyapatite. Since bone induction mediated by the influence of degrading bone matrix on non-specific mesenchymal cells is a known effect, but did not occur in our tests with hydroxyapatite, one is led to assume that in principle two different forms of osteoinduction are possible: (a) osteoinduction by bone morphogenetic protein; (b) stimulation and induction of osteoprogenitor cells, as in apatite implantation. Burchardt (1983) used the term "osteoconduction" for this stimulation of bone regeneration in beds with high regenerative capacity. In order to avoid misunderstanding we have used the designation "osteoconduction or osteostimulation" for bone-stimulating effects in beds of high regenerative capacity. The term "osteoconductive" is yet misleading, since the stimulation of osteogenesis with Pyrost or Collapat involves not just serving as a scaffold for the formation of new bone but, above all, a quantitatively measurable increase in the amount of new bone growth. In this context, the hypothesis put forward by Friedenstein (1973) should be highlighted. Friedenstein assumed that two separate colonies of osteoprogenitor cells exist. He termed these colonies "determined" and "inducible" osteogenic precursor cells. The determined osteoprogenitor cells may not be only conducted by mineral bone and hydroxy apatite granules but also be biologically stimulated.

The results of our experiments leave several questions unanswered. First of all, it needs to be established whether the massive stimulation of bone regeneration seen with hydroxyapatite in its different application forms in rabbits can be reproduced in another species, e.g. in the dog. Furthermore, we performed all our experiments with beds of high regenerative capacity, so that at present Collapat E and Pyrost can only be recommended for use in those defects. Further tests in beds of low regenerative capacity are therefore required. Muscle-implantation experiments that have since been performed by W. Mittelmeier showed no bone induction with Pyrost alone, but upon concurrent administration of bone-marrow cells intense formation of new bone was observed in beds of low regenerative capacity as well.

As mentioned earlier in the general discussion of Collapat and Pyrost (Sect. 4.6 and Sect. 4.8), clinical tests have already begun on both preparations, and over 250 Collapat implantations and more than 350 Pyrost implantations in man have already been made in our university. Clinically we feel that these bone substitutes are very helpful for reconstruction of certain bone defects. In bigger defects these bone substitutes are used either as augmentation material of autografts or combined with autogenous bone marrow.

If the observed effects of Collapat and Pyrost should be re-confirmed in the further investigations which are planned, then promising new techniques for local bone regeneration with these bone-replacement materials will open up in reconstructive surgery for bone defects of various types, and help to avoid the draw-backs of autogenic, allogenic and xenogenic bone transplants. In future, this development will probably lead to a reduction in transplantation of autografts and allografts.

7 Summary

After an initial review of bone biology, the "state of the art" in the different bone-transplantation techniques has been presented in detail. The superior efficacy of autogenic spongiosa has been highlighted, but its problems and disadvantages have also been discussed. Allogenic bone transplants are characterised by immuno-defensive reactions, but allow creeping substitution and osteoconduction, and are therefore used in several clinics as an alternative to autogenic bone transplants. Besides the immuno-defensive reaction, an important disadvantage of this technique is the considerable resources required for the operation of a carefully managed bone bank. Since the beginning of this decade skeletal allografting has become more popular. The results of osteochondral allograft resurfacing, allografts in tumour surgery and revision hip arthroplasty are encouraging. However resorption, fractures and the risk of disease transfer are considerable problems. Because of even stronger immuno-defensive reactions, xenogenic bone transplants are no longer in use today.

The principal objective of this project was the study of so-called bone-replacement materials. These have been introduced in a detailed literature survey. Our own animal experiments with different bone-replacement materials have been presented, and the regenerated bone was been evaluated histomorphometrically where possible.

In the course of this project, 168 tests on 84 rabbits were performed. Since a sophisticated un-decalcified bone histology technique is a pre-requisite for bone histomorphometry, an introduction to our own histological technique has been given. In a total of 32 control experiments we have shown that, even in the spongy recipient bed of the rabbit, spontaneous bone regeneration has its limits, and untreated 6 mm drilled cavity defects persist for a long period.

In agreement with published literature, we found that transplanted autogenic spongiosa is rapidly incorporated into the bone defect and induces further osteoregeneration.

So-called bone matrix (BMP) has been proven by numerous authors to induce bone regeneration in heterotopic sites. Unfortunately this material is not yet available for clinical practice. In our experiments bone matrix does occasionally exhibit bone growth on its surface, but it is not possible to show a statistically significant quantitative difference in induction of bone regeneration in comparison to empty cavities. Recently, Urist et al. (1984) also recommended mixing bone matrix (BMP) with tricalcium phosphate, which results in 12 times more bone formation than without tricalcium phosphate. The extraction of pure "osteogenin" remains to be seen.

After a latency period, Kiel bone splinters induce a strong defensive reaction, which attacks not only the transplant but also the regenerated bone. The inadequacy of Kiel bone splinters is explained by the immuno-defensive reaction they induce due to incomplete deproteination of the collagenous structures.

Various gelatin preparations (from Merck and Riedel) did not induce any inflammatory defensive reactions, but promotion of bone growth could not be detected with these implantation materials.

While a mixture of collagen web and apatite powder did not convincingly promote bone regeneration, ceramised apatite granules stimulated intensive bone regeneration on their surfaces without inducing the formation of separating connective-tissue layer or provoking any defensive reactions at all. However, the apatite granules used initially were too large; also, they were not evenly distributed within the defect cavity, due to sedimentation and washing out.

Therefore, smaller ceramised apatite granules were used in the subsequent experiments and were embedded in a collagen web. Later, the collagen web was given additional structural stability by cross-linking. The final development stage produced a product which was designated "Collapat E", and which consists of small ceramised apatite granules as the principal osteoregenerative components, mixed and finely dispersed with a purified and further cross-linked collagen web (as carrier) in a ratio of 5:1. Histomorphometric evaluation of our animal experiments showed that this product permits excellent realisation of Mittelmeier's conception of multi-centric bone regeneration around dispersed hydroxyapatite particles in orthotopic sites. In comparison with empty cavities, statistically significant promotion of bone growth (on average 4.5 times more bone formation) is obtained. In comparison with autogenic spongiosa, the rate of bone regeneration with this product is not significantly different.

Further studies were made with a totally deproteinated mineral bone (Pyrost), obtained by pyrolysis and sintering, that also stimulated rapid and complete bone regeneration. In this respect, this mineral bone is superior to the synthetic porous hydroxyapatite ceramic materials which, in pilot experiments, also showed good bone regeneration on their surface, but did not lead to complete bridging of the defect cavity with regenerated bone. When using either Collapat or Pyrost in recipient beds of low regenerative capacity, it is necessary also to administer osteogenic cells (spongiosa or bone marrow) at the same time, because these bone substitutes are not osteoinductive.

The mode of action of both Collapat and Pyrost is osteostimulation by osteoconduction. The determined osteoprogenitor cells in the implant bed may not only be conducted but also be biologically stimulated. This biological stimulation by calcium phosphates is probably the same phenomenon which has been observed by Urist et al. (1984) in the above-mentioned combination of BMP with tricalcium phosphate. BMP is part of the bone and must be present in the area surrounding any bone defect, as in our own experimental set-up. BMP and ceramic hydroxyapatite or β-tricalcium phosphate may act together in the multifactorial process of bone regeneration.

Our own experimental results prove that hydroxyapatite in an appropriate application, which does not hinder bone in growth by abundant material at the same time, quantitatively stimulates bone regeneration. By this the principle of osteoconduction has proven to be significant.

Hydroxyapatite and tricalcium phosphate will undoubtedly find a place in bone surgery due to their outstanding bioactivity and biocompatibility, not only as bone substitutes but also as a coating material for implants.

We have used both Collapat and Pyrost in clinical trials at our university with over 700 patients. In appropriate indications they are very helpful and effective bone substitutes.

References

Abbott LC, Schottstaedt ER, Saunders JB, Dec M, Bost FC (1947) The evaluation of cortical and cancellous bone as grafting material. J Bone Joint Surg 29:381
Abbott WM, Austen WG (1974) Microcrystalline collagen as hemostatic agent for vascular surgery. Surgery 76:291
Abbott WM, Austen WG (1975) The effectiveness and mechanism of collagen-induced topical hemostasis. Surgery 78:723
Ackermann W, Taillard W (1977) Transplantation von konservierter, homogener Spongiosa. Z Orthop 115:679
Aebi M, Regazzoni P (1987) Bone transplantation, up-dating on osteochondral auto- and allografting. Springer, Berlin Heidelberg New York Tokyo (to be published)
Albee FH, Morrison HF (1920) Studies in bone growth triple calcium phosphate as a stimules to osteogenesis. Ann Surg 71:32
Albrektsson T, Lindner L (1981) Intravital, long-term follow-up of autologous experimental bone grafts. Arch Orthop Traumat Surg 98:189
Algire GH, Weaver GM, Prehn RT (1954) Growth of cells "in vivo" in diffusion chambers survival in homograft in immunized mice. J Natl Cancer Inst 15:493
Anderson HC (1969) Vesicles associated with calcification in the matrix of epiphyseal cartilage. J Cell Biol 41:59
Arnold IS, Frost HM, Buss RO (1971) The osteocyte as a bone pump. Clin Orthop 78:47
Axhausen G (1908) Die pathologisch-anatomischen Grundlagen der Lehre von der freien Knochentransplantation beim Menschen und beim Tier. Med Klin 2:23
Axhausen W (1952) Die Knochenregeneration – ein zweiphasisches Geschehen. Zentralbl Chir 11:435
Balleisen L, Gay S, Marx R, Kühn K (1975) Comparative investigation on the influence of human bovine collagen types I, II and II on the aggregation of human platelets. Klin Wochenschr 53:903
Bassett CAL (1966) Electro-mechanical factors regulating bone architecture. In: Flinch H, Blackwood HJJ, Owen M (eds) Third Symposium on Calcified Tissues. Springer, Berlin Heidelberg New York
Bassett CAL, Hurley LA, Stinchfield FE (1962) The fate of long-term anorganic bone implants. Transplantation 29:423–451
Bauermeister A (1958) Experimentelle Grundlagen für den Aufbau einer neuen Knochenbank. Hefte Unfallheilkd 58
Bauermeister A (1961) Die Behandlung von Zysten, Tumoren und entzündlichen Prozessen des Knochens mit dem „Kieler Knochenspan". Bruns Beitr Klin Chir 203:287
Bedacht R (1969) Tierexperimentelle und klinische Untersuchungen über die Anwendung von heterologem Kollagen als Implantat in der Knochenhöhle von Röhrenknochen. Habilitationsschrift, Universität München
Belanger LF (1971) Osteocytic resorption. In: Bowae GH (ed) The biochemistry and physiology of bone. Academic Press, New York
Benfer J, Struck H (1972) Förderung der Frakturheilung durch lokale Kollagenapplikation. Dtsch Med Wochenschr 97:523
Bhaskar SN, Brady JM, Getter L, Grower MF, Driskell T (1971) Biodegradable ceramic implants in bone. Oral Surg 32:336
Blechschmidt E (1960) Die vorgeburtlichen Entwicklungsstadien des Menschen. Karger, Basel Freiburg London New York
Blencke BA, Brömer H, Deutscher K (1975) Glaskeramik – ein neuer, bioaktiver Implantatwerkstoff. Med Orthop Techn 95:144
Blencke BA, Brömer H, Deutscher K (1980) The adhesion of loaded glass-ceramic implants to bone. In: Hastings GW, Williams DF (eds) Mechanical properties of biomaterials. Wiley & Sons, New York Chichester

Boellaard JW, Hirsch T von (1959) Die Herstellung histologischer Schnitte von nicht entkalktem Knochen mittels Einbettung in Methacrylsäureester. Mikroskopie 13:186
Bösch P, Litner F, Artes H, Brand G (1980) Experimental investigations of the effect of the fibrin adhesive on the Kiel heterologous bone graft. Arch Orthop Trauma Surg 96:177
Bonfiglio M, Jeter WS (1972) Immunological responses to bone. Clin Orthop 87:19
Bonucci E (1976) Fine structure of early cartilage calcification. J Ultrastruct Res 20:33
Borckmann BU, Frenkel G, Hauk H (1982) Knochenheilung nach Gelatineschwammimplantation unter Kompression beim Hund. Dtsch Zahnärztl Z 37:25
Bordier PJ, Tun Chot S (1972) Quantitative histology of metabolic bone disease. Clin Endocrinol Metab 1:197
Boskey AL (1981) Current concepts of the physiology and biochemistry of calcification. Clin Orthop 157:225
Boutin P (1972) Arthroplastie totale de la hanche par prothese en alumine fritee. Rev Chir Orthop 58:229
Brill W, Katthagen BD (1987) Die Grenzschicht zwischen Hydroxylapatit-Keramik und neugebildetem Knochen im Rasterelektronenmikroskop. Z Orthop 125:183
Brown WE, Chow LC (1976) Chemical properties of bone mineral. Ann Rev Muter Sci 6:213
Bulletin Synthes (1983) Neuheiten und Modifikationen im Originalinstrumentarium der Arbeitsgemeinschaft für Osteosynthesefragen (AO). „Ceros 80" Nr. 52 3.83 Bulletin Synthes
Burchardt H (1983) The biology of bone graft repair. Clin Orthop 174:28
Burchardt H, Busbee III GA, Enneking WF (1975) Repair of experimental autologous grafts of cortical bone. J Bone Joint Surg (Am) 57:814
Burchardt H, Jones H, Glowczewskie F, Rudener C, Enneking WF (1978) Freeze dried allogenic segmental cortical bone grafts in dogs. J Bone Joint Surg (Am) 60:1032
Burkhardt R (1966a) Präoperative Voraussetzungen zur klinischen Histologie des menschlichen Knochenmarks. Blut 13:337
Burkhardt R (1966b) Präoperative Voraussetzungen zur klinischen Histologie des menschlichen Knochenmarks. Blut 14:30
Burri C (1979) Posttraumatische Osteitis, 2. Aufl. Huber, Bern Stuttgart Wien
Burri C, Henkmeyer H, Rüedi T (1971) Chirurgische Behandlung infizierter Knochendefekte. Langenbecks Arch Chir 330:54
Carter DR, Spengler DM (1978) Mechanical properties and composition of cortical bone. Clin Orthop 135:192
Chacha PB (1984) Vascularized pedicular bone grafts. Int Orthop 8:117
Chalmers J (1959) Transplantation immunity in bone homografting. J Bone Joint Surg (Br) 41:160
Chalmers J, Gray DH, Rush J (1975) Observations of the suduction of bone in soft tissues. J Bone Joint Surg (Br) 57:36
Chvapil M, Holusa R (1968) Experimental experience with the collagen sponge as hemostypticum and tampon. J Biomed Mater Res 2:1
Chvapil M, Krajicek M (1967) Die Analyse einiger theoretischer Probleme bei der Verwendung von Erzeugnissen aus Kollagen in der Medizin. Langenbecks Arch Klin Chir 318:80
Clark JH (1931) A study of tendons, bones and other forms of connective tissue by means of X-ray diffraction patterns. Ann J Physiol 98:328
Clarke WJ, Driskell T, Hassler CR, Tennery VJ, McCoy LR (1973) Calcium phosphate resorbable ceramics: A potential alternative to bone grafting (Abstracts). IADR 5 1st General Meeting Chicago, p 259
Cobb CM, Howell BE, Gray RC, Weatherford TW (1976) Potential of elastin and collagen as initiators of in vivo calcification. Oral Surg 41:24
Cutright DE, Bhaskar SN, Brady JM, Getter L, Posey WR (1972) Reaction of bone to tricalcium phosphate ceramic pellets. Oral Surg 33:850
Cutright DE, Posey WR, Bhaskar SN, Larson WJ (1973) Collagen sponge subcutaneous implantation. Oral Surg 35:144
Dahmen G, Koch W (1962) Histologische Untersuchungen über den Ein- und Umbau heterologer macerierter Knochenimplantate. Arch Orthop Unfallchir 54:139
Dambe LT, Saur K, Schweiberer L (1978) Revaskularisation frischer homologer Knochentransplantate in der Diaphyse des Röhrenknochens beim Hund. Arch Orthop Trauma Aurg 92:35
Daume E (1982) Lokale Blutstillung, Gynäkologie und Geburtshilfe. In: Breddin HK, Siewert JR (Hrsg) Lokale Blutstillung. Bibliomedizinische Verl Ges, Melsungen

Decker S, Müller KH (1980) Morphologisch-experimentelle Untersuchungen über die vom Lager ausgehende Vascularisation autologer Spongiosatransplantate. In: Hierholzer G, Zilch H (Hrsg) Transplantatlager und Implantatlager bei verschiedenen Operationsverfahren. Springer, Berlin Heidelberg New York, S 32

Decker S, Müller-Färber J, Decker B (1979) Die Knochenneubildung im autologen Spongiosatransplantat - morphologisch-experimentelle Untersuchung. Z Plast Chir 3/3:159

Delling G (1974) Altersabhängige Skelettveränderungen. Klin Wochenschr 52:318

Denissen HW, de Groot K, Makkes PC, van den Hooff A, Klopper PJ (1980) Tissue response to dense apatite implants in rats. J Biomed Mater Res 14:713

Dixon TF, Perkins HR (1956) The chemistry of calcification. In: Bourne GH (ed) The biochemistry ad physiology of bone. Academic Press, New York

Doty SB, Schofield BH (1972) Electron microscopic localization of hydrolytic enzymes in osteoclasts. Histochem J 4:245

Driessen AA, Klein CPAT, de Groot K (1982) Preparation and some properties of sintered β-whitlockite. Biomaterials 3:113

Ecke H (1967) Neue Wege der quantitativen Bestimmung der ossären Regeneration an Knochentransplantaten. Langenbecks Arch Chir 319:448

Ecke H (1976) Der Kompakta-Test im Spiegel früherer und neuerer Ergebnisse. Unfallchirurgie 2:91

Eger W (1963) Kalziumnachweis und Mineralisation des Knochengewebes. Verhandlungen der Deutschen Gesellschaft für Pathologie. 47. Tagung. Fischer, Stuttgart, S 54

Eger W, Götz F, Kämmerer H (1964) Herstellung von Dünnschliffen aus Knochen und Weichgewebe nach Markierung mit Tetracyclinen. Langenbecks Arch Chir 306:205

Ehalt W (1968) Hat die Knochenbank noch ihre Berechtigung? Arch Orthop Unfallchir 64:1

Eisen E (1979) Methyl-Methacrylat-Einbettung, Schneiden und Färben unentkalkter Knochen-Kompakta. MTA 4:147

Eitel F, Seiler H, Schweiberer L (1981) Vergleichende morphologische Untersuchungen zur Übertragbarkeit tierexperimenteller Ergebnisse auf den Regenerationsprozeß des menschlichen Röhrenknochens. Unfallheilkd 84:250, 255

Elliott JC (1973) The problems of the composition and structure of the mineral components of the hard tissues. Clin Orthop 93:313

Ellis HA, Peart KM (1972) Quantitative observations on mineralized and nonmineralized bone in the iliac crest. J Clin Pathol 25:277

Elves MW (1978) Cell mediated immunity to allografts of fresh and treated bone. Int Orthop 2:171

Elves MW, Salama R (1974) A study of the development of cytotoxic antibodies produced in recipients of xenografts (heterografts) of iliac bone. J Bone Joint Surg (Br) 56:331

Engström A (1946) Quantitative micro- and histochemical elementary analysis. Acta Radiol (Suppl) 63:1

Engström A (1963) Physikalische Methoden zur Untersuchung des Knochengewebes. Verhandlungen der Deutschen Gesellschaft für Pathologie, 47. Tagung. Fischer, Stuttgart, S 15

Enneking WF (1962) Immunologic aspects of bone transplantation. South Med J 55:894

Eriksson C, Jones S (1977) Bone mineral and serface charge. Clin Orthp 128:351

Eulenberger J, Stich H, Niederer PG (1978) Biokeramik im Rattenversuch. Schweiz Monatsschr Zahnheilkd 88:378

Fabinger A, Krekeler G, Vogel D (1980) Anwendungsmöglichkeiten von Kollagen zur parodontalen Knochentasche. Dtsch Zahnärztl Z 35:9

Ferraro J, Foreman D (1978) Analysis of Ca_3 $(pO_4)2$ bone implant in ilium canis to assess resorption (Abstracts). IADR 67 General Meeting New Orleans, 1278

Fincato M (1982) Abdominalchirurgie. In: Breddin HK, Siewert JR (Hrsg) Lokale Blutstillung. Bibliomed, Melsungen

Fischer E (1971) Meeting on ethylene oxide sterilisation. University Hospital of Wales

Flatley TJ, Lynch KL, Benson M (1983) Tissue response to implants of calcium phosphate ceramic in the rabbit spine. Clin Orthop 179:246

Fleisch H, Neuman WF (1961) Mechanism of calcification – role of collagen, polyphosphates and phosphates. Am J Physiol 200:1296

Forgon M, Bornemisza G (1970) Über die Revaskularisierung eines auto- und homoioplastischen Spongiosatransplantates im Tierversuch. Bruns Beitr Klin Chir 218:277

Freitag V, Ruppersberg H (1972) Kontaktmikroradiographie verkalkter biologischer Objekte mit charakteristischer Röntgen-Strahlung. Dtsch Zahnärztl Z 27:749

Freitag V, Stetter W (1973) Röntgenröhre für die Kontaktmikroradiographie verkalkter biologischer Objekte. Röntgenblätter 7:289
Friedebold G, Witt AN, Hanslik L, Jendryschik A (1963) Kritische Untersuchungen über den klinischen Wert homoio- und heterologer Knochentransplantation. Arch Orthop Unfallchir 55:627
Friedenstein AJ (1973) Determined and inducable osteogenic precursor cells. In: Hard tissue growth repair and remineralization. Ciba Foundation Symposium Elsevier. Excerpta-Medica, Amsterdam, p 169
Friedenstein AJ, Lalykina KS, Tolmacheva AA (1967) Osteogenic activity of peritoneal fluid cells induced by transitional epithelium. Acta Anat (Basel) 68:532
Friedenstein AJ, Petrakova KV, Kurolesova AJ, Frolova GP (1968) Heterotopic transplants of bone marrow. Analysis of precursor cells for osteogenic and haematopoietic tissuese. Transplantation 6:230
Friedlaender GE (1983) Bone and cartilage transplantation. Clin Orthop 174:2
Friedlaender GE, Mankin HJ, Sell KW (eds) (1983) Osteochondral allografts. Little Brown, Boston
Frost HM (1961) Tetracycline labeling of bone and the zone of demarcation of osteoid seams. Can J Biochem 40:485
Frost HM (1964) Dynamics of bone remodeling. In: Frost HM (ed) Bone biodynamics. Little Brown, Boston Massachusetts, p 315
Frost HM (1966) The bone biodynamics in osteoporosis and osteomalacia. Thomas, Springfield
Fuchs GA (1983) Glaskeramik als bioaktiver Implantatwerkstoff für belastete Gelenkimplantate im Tierexperiment. Habilitationsschrift, Universität Marburg
Funovics JM, Seidl W, Polterauer P (1982) Fibrin-Kollagen-Klebung in der Abdominalchirurgie mit besonderer Berücksichtigung der Leberresektion. In: Breddin HK, Siewert JR (Hrsg) Lokale Blutstillung. Bibliomed, Melsungen
Gelhar P (1980) Die Osteonenausmessung – ein neues Verfahren zur Auswertung von Knochenpräparaten in der Fluoreszenzmikroskopie. Inaugural-Dissertation, Universität Düsseldorf
Getter L, Bhaskar SM, Cutright DE, Perez B, Brady JM, Driskel TD, O'Hara MJ (1972) Three biodegradable calcium phosphate slurry implants in bone. J Oral Surg 30:263
Gewalt R, Fischer E (1959) Ein neues Gerät zur Sterilisation mit gespanntem Äthylenoxyd. Münch Med Wochenschr 13:563
Glowacki J, Kaban LB, Murray JE, Folkman J, Mulliken JB (1981) Application of the biological principle of induced osteogenesis for craniofacial defects. Lancet 1:959
Graf R (1959) Gefäßversorgung alloplastischer Spongiosatransplantate und ihre Bedeutung. Bruns Beitr Klin Chir 198:390
Griss P, Krempien B, Andrian-Werburg H, von Heimke G, Fleiner R (1973) Experimentelle Untersuchungen zur Gewebeverträglichkeit oxidkeramischer Abriebteile. Arch Orthop Unfallchir 76:270
Gross A, McKee N, Farine I, Czitrom A, Langer F (1984) Reconstruction of skeletal defects following enbloc excision of bone tumours. In: Uhthoff HK (ed) Current concept of diagnosis and treatment of bone and soft tissue tumours. Springer, Berlin Heidelberg New York Tokyo
Gück U (1957) Über vergleichende histologische und röntgenologische Untersuchungen an menschlichem Knochengewebe. RÖFO 86:728
Hait MR, Robb CA, Baxter CR, Borgmann AR, Tippett LO (1973) Comparative evaluation of avitane microcrystalline collagen hermostat in experimental animal wounds. Am J Surg 125:284
Haldeman KO, Moore JM (1934) Influence of a local excess of calcium and phosphorus on the healing of fractures. Arch Surg 29:385
Hancox NH (1972) Biology of bone. Cambridge University Press, Cambridge
Harakas NK (1984) Demineralized bone-matrix-induced osteogenesis. Clin Orthop 188:239
Harms J, Mäusle E (1980) Biokompatibilität von Implantaten in der Orthopädie. Hefte Unfallheilkd 144. Springer, Berlin Heidelberg New York
Harper RA, Posner AS (1966) Measurement of non-crystalline calcium phosphate in bone mineral. Proc Soc Exp Biol 122:137
Harris WH (1960) A microscope method of determining rates of bone growth. Nature 188:1038
Harris WH, Jackson RH, Jowsey J (1962) The in vivo distribution of tetracyclines in canine bone. J Bone Joint Surg (Am) 44:1308
Harris WH, Lavorgna J, Hamblen DL, Haywood EA (1968) The inhibition of ossification in vivo. Clin Orthop 61:52

Haussmann P, Mergard UE, Köhnlein HE (1974) Zur Wirkung verschiedener Hämostyptica. Fortschr Med 92:579
Hayashi K, Yabuki T, Tabuchi K, Fujii T (1982) Repair of experimental bone defect with a collagen block containing synthesized apatit. Arch Orthop Trauma Surg 99:265
Hayek E (1967) Die Mineralsubstanz der Knochen. Klin Wochenschr 17:857
Heiple KG, Chase SW, Herndon CH (1963) A comparative study of the healing process following different types of bone transplantation. J Bone Joint Surg (Am) 45:1593
Hench LL (1975) Ceramic implants. Glass Ceram Bull 22:82
Hench LL (1980) The interfacial behaviour of biomaterials. J Biomed Mater Res 14:803
Hench LL, Splinter RJ, Allen C, Greenle TK (1971) Bonding mechanisms at the interface of ceramic prosthetic materials. J Biomed Mater REs 2/1:117
Henschke F, Pesch HJ (1978) Kunststoffeinbettung im Knochenlabor. Präparative Voraussetzungen zur Schnitt- und Schlifftechnik. MTA 5:211
Hirsch T von, Boellard JW (1958) Methacrylsäureester als Einbettungsmittel in der Histologie. Z Wiss Mikrosk 64:24
Hörmann H (1967) Untereinheiten und Quervernetzungen im Kollagen. Leder 18:215
Holmes RE (1979) Bone regeneration within a coralline hydroxylapatite implant. Plast Reconstr Surg 63:626
Holmstrand K (1967) Biophysical investigations of bone transplants and bone implants. Acta Orthop Scand (Suppl) 26
Holtrop ME, Weinger JM (1972) Ultrastructural evidence for a transport system in bone. In: Talmage RV, Munson DL (eds) Parathyroid hormone and the calcitonins. International Congress Series No 243. Excerpta Medica, Amsterdam
Hopf A (1957) Diskussionsbemerkung. Verh Dtsch Ges Orthop 90:440
Hovig T, Jorgensen L, Packham MA, Mustard JF (1968) Platelet adherance to fibrin and collagen. J Lab Clin Med 71:29
Huggins CB (1930) Influence of the urinary tract mucosa on the experimental formation of bone. Proc Soc Exp Biol Med 27:349
Hunt LM, Benoit PW (1976) Evaluation of a microcrystalline collage preparation in extraction wounds. J Oral Surg 34:407
Irving JT (1973) Theories of mineralization of bone. Clin Orthop 97:225
Irving JT, Wuthier RE (1968) Histochemistry and biochemistry of calcification with special reference to the role of lipids. Clin Orthop 56:237
Jahn TL (1968) A possible mechanism for the effect of electrical potentials on apatite formation in bone. Clin Orthop 56:261
Jande SS, Belanger LF (1973) The life cycle of the osteocyte. Clin Orthop 94:281
Jarcho M (1981) Calcium phosphate ceramics as hard tissue prosthetics. Clin Orthop 157:259
Jarcho M, Bolen CH, Thomas MB, Bobick J, Kay JF, Doremus RH (1976) Hydroxylapatite synthesis and characterization in dense polycrystalline form. J Mater Sci 11:2027
Jarcho M, Kay JF, Gumaer KI, Doremus RH, Drobeck HP (1977) Tissue, cellular and subcellular events at a bone-ceramic hydroxylapatite interface.
Joos U, Ochs G (1979) Einfluß von gelöstem heterologen Kollagen auf die Aggregation menschlicher Thrombozyten. Dtsch Zahnärztl Z 34:35
Joos U, Ochs G (1980) Heterologes Kollagen als Kristallisationskeim für die Knochenmineralisation. Dtsch Zahnärztl Z 35:2
Joos U, Vogel D, Ries P (1979) Die Verwendung von Kollagenvlies zum Auffüllen von Knochendefekten in der Kiefer-Gesichts-Chirurgie. Dtsch Z Mund-Kiefer-Gesichtschir 3:104
Jowsey J, Kelly PJ, Riggs BL, Bianco AJ, Scholz DA, Gershon-Cohen J (1965) Quantitative microradiographic studies of normal and osteoporotic bone. J Bone Joint Surg (Am) 47:785
Kaiser G, Wagner W, Tetuh P, Köster K (1980) Zur Regeneration knöcherner Defekte nach der Implantation resorbierbarer Kalziumphosphatkeramik. Eine vergleichende klinische Untersuchung. Dtsch Zahnärztl Z 35:108
Kallenberger A (1978) Die Wirkung von Biokeramik (Kalziumphosphatkeramik) auf kultivierte Kaninchenfibroblasten. Schweiz Monatsschr Zahnheilkd 88:90–112
Karlson P (1972) Kurzes Lehrbuch der Biochemie. Thieme, Stuttgart
Katthagen BD, Bechtel U (1985) Technik der unentkalkten Knochenhistologie und Histomorphometrie. MTA-Journal 7:164

Katthagen BD, Hellstern P (1984) In vitro-Untersuchungen über die Wirkung von gelöstem und ungelöstem heterologen Collagen-Vlies auf menschliche Thrombozyten. Z Orthop 122:677
Katthagen BD, Mittelmeier H (1983a) Eine neue quantitative Methode in der experimentellen Knochenhistologie. Vortrag D.G.O.T. Essen
Katthagen BD, Mittelmeier H (1983b) Vergleichende tierexperimentelle Untersuchungen über die induktive Knochenregeneration mit pyrolisiertem enteiweißtem Knochenimplantat. Vortrag Dtsch Ges Plast Whst Chir, Gießen
Katthagen BD, Mittelmeier H (1984) Experimental animal investigation of bone regeneration with collagen apatite. Arch Orthop Trauma Surg 103:291
Kember NF (1960) Cell division in enchondral ossification. J Bone Joint Surg (Br) 42:824
Kim KM (1976) Calcification of matrix resides in human aortic valve and aortic media. Fed Proc 35:156
Klawitter JJ, Hulbert SF (1972) Application of porous ceramics for the attachment of load beaving internal orthopedic applications. J Biomed Mater Res 2/1:161
Knese KH (1959) Die Ultrastruktur des Knochengewebes. Dtsch Med Wochenschr 84:1640
Knöfler EW (1976) Ergebnisse der homologen Knochentransplantation. Nova Acta Leopoldina 44:413
Knöfler EW (1978) Die Knochenbank der Orthopädischen Klinik der Karl-Marx-Universität Leipzig. Beitr Orthop Traumatol 25:72
Köhnlein HE, Mergard U (1972) Experimentelle Testung lokaler Hämostyptica. Chirurg 43:378
Köster K, Karbe E, Kramer H, Heide H, König R (1976) Experimenteller Knochenersatz durch resorbierbare Calciumphosphat-Keramik. Langenbecks Arch Chir 341:77
Köster K, Heide H, König R (1977) Resorbiere Calciumphosphatkeramik im Tierexperiment unter Belastung. Langenbecks Arch Chir 343:173
Köster K, Ehard H, Kubicek J, Heide H (1979) Experimentelle Anwendung von Kalziumphosphatgranulat zur Substitution von konventionellen Knochentransplantaten. Z Orthop 118:398
Koskinen EVS, Salenius P, Alho A (1979) Allogenic transplantation in low-grade malignant bone tumours. Acta Orthop Scand 50:129
Krekeler G, Düker J, Fabinger A (1980) Tierexperimentelle Untersuchungen zur Knochenregeneration nach Implantation heteroplastischer Materialien. Dtsch Zahnärztl Z 35:5
Krempien B (1982) Mineralisation und Verkalkung unter normalen und pathologischen Bedingungen. In: Ziegler R (Hrsg) EHDP Ein neues therapeutisches Prinzip bei Osteopathien und Calciumstoffwechselstörungen. Urban & Schwarzenberg, München Wien Baltimore
Krempien B, Lemminger FM, Ritz E, Weber E (1978) The reaction of different skeletal sites to metabolic bone disease – A micromorphometric study. Klin Wochenschr 56:755
Krompecher S (1937) Die Knochenbildung. Fischer, Jena
Kropp BM (1954) Grinding thin sections of plastic-embedded bone. Stain Technol. 29:77
Kühn K, Zimmer E (1961) Eigenschaften des Tropokollagenmoleküls und deren Bedeutung für die Fibrillenbildung. Z Naturforsch 16b:648
Langer F, Czitrom A, Pritzker KP, Gross AE (1975) The immunigenicity of fresh and frozen allogeneic bone. J Bone Joint Surg (Am) 57:216
Lentz W (1955) Die Grundlagen der Transplantation von fremdem Knochengewebe. Thieme, Stuttgart
Levitt SJ, Crayton PH, Monroe EA, Condrate RA (1969) Forming methods for apatite prosthesis. J Biomed Mater Res 3:683
Lexer E (1911) Über freie Transplantationen. Langenbecks Arch Chir 95:827
Locht RC, Gross AE, Langer F (1984) Late ostechondral allograft resurfacing for tibial plateau fractures. J Bone Joint Surg (Am) 66:328
Lowe J, Stein H, Sela J (1983) Primary calcification in remodeling haverian systems following tibial fracture in rats. Clin Orthop 176:291
Maatz R (1959) Klinische Erfahrungen mit dem eiweißarmen Tierspan. Langenbecks Arch Chir 292:831
Maatz R, Bauermeister A (1961) 36. Klinische Erfahrungen mit dem Kieler Span. Langenbecks Arch Chir 298:239
Maatz R, Lentz W, Graf R (1952) Die Knochenbildungsfähigkeit konservierter Späne. Ein Beitrag zur Knochenbank. Zentralbl Chir 77:1376
Maatz R, Lentz W, Graf R (1954) Spongiosatest of bone grafts. J Bone Joint Surg (Am) 36:721
Marchand F (1899) Zur Kenntnis der Knochentransplantation. Verh Dtsch Ges Pathol, S 368
Matti H (1932) Über freie Transplantation von Knochenspongiosa. Langenbecks Arch Chir 168:236
Medawar PB (1944) The behavious and fate of skin autografts and skin homografts in rabbits. J Anat 78:176

Melsen F, Melsen B, Mosekilde L (1978) An evaluation of the quantitative parameters applied in bone histology. Acta Pathol Microbiol Immunol Scand (A) 86:63
Menzel J, Steffen C (1974) Immunogenicity and speciticity of collagen. Immunology 26:417
Merz WA (1967) Die Streckenmessung an gerichteten Strukturen im Mikroskop und ihre Anwendung zur Bestimmung von Oberflächen-Volumen-Relationen im Knochengewebe. Mikroskopie 22:132
Merz WA, Schenk RK (1970) A quantitative histological study on bone formation in human cancellous bone. Acta Anat 76:1
Milch RA, Rall DP, Tobie JE (1958) Fluorescence of tetracycline antibiotics in bone. J Bone Joint Surg (Am) 40:897
Miller EJ (1973) A review of biochemical studies on the genetically distinct collagens of the skeletal system. Clin Orthop 92:260
Mittelmeier H (1974) Zementlose Verankerung von Endoprothesen nach dem Tragrippenprinzip. Z Orthop 112:27
Mittelmeier H (1984) Hüftgelenkersatz bei jungen Menschen. Z Orthop 122:20
Mittelmeier H, Katthagen BD (1983) Klinische Erfahrungen mit Collagen-Apatit-Implantation zur lokalen Knochenregeneration. Z Orthop 121:115
Mittelmeier H, Katthagen BD (1984) Neue Wege des Knochenersatzes. Orthop Prax 20:389
Mittelmeier H, Nizard M (1982) Knochenregeneration mit industriell gefertigtem Collagen-Apatit-Implantat. In: Hackenbroch MH, Refior HJ, Jäger M (Hrsg) Osteogenese und Knochenwachstum. Thieme, Stuttgart New York
Mittelmeier H, Nizard M (1983) Kollagenvlies mit Apatit als künstliches Knochenersatzmaterial auf natürlicher Basis. In: Kley W, Naumann C (Hrsg) Regionale plastische und rekonstruktive Chirurgie im Kindesalter (Vortrag 1981). Springer, Berlin Heidelberg New York
Mittelmeier H, Hanser U, Harms J (1980) Zur Lösung des Zementproblems mittels Apatit-Carbonfaser-Knochenzement. Z Orthop 118:658
Mittelmeier W (in Vorbereitung) Knochenregeneration im ersatzschwachen Lager mit und ohne autologe Markinokulation. Inauguraldissertation Homburg
Monroe EA, Votava W, Bass DB, McMullen J (1971) New calcium phosphate ceramic material for bone and tooth implants. J Dent Res 50:860
Moore MAS, Metcalf D (1970) Ontogeny of the haemoprietic systems: Yolk sac origin in vivo and in vitro colony forming cells in the developing mouse embryo. Br J Haematol 18:279
Müller KH (1981) Exogene Osteomyelitis von Becken und unteren Gliedmaßen. Springer, Berlin Heidelberg New York
Münzenberg KJ (1970) Untersuchungen zur Kristallographie der Knochenminerale. Biomineralisation 1:67
Najarian JS (1962) Mechanism of homograft rejection. Plast Reconstr Surg 39:359
Narang R, Wells H (1973) Experimental osteogenesis in periapical areas with decalcified allogeneic bone matrix. Oral Surg 35:136
Needleman SB, Stefanovic N (1969) Production of antibody for rat tail tendon collagen. Experientia 25:1335
Neuberger A (1955) Metabolism of collagen under normal conditions. In: Fibrous proteins and their biological significance. Symp Soc Expl Biol No 9. Cambridge University Press, Cambridge
Newseley H, Osborn JF (1978) Structural and textural implications of calcium phosphates in ceramics. III. Conference on materials for use in medicine and biology bioceramics symposium Keele University, Sept 1978
Niwa S, Sawai K, Takahashi S, Tagai H, Ono M, Fukuda Y (1980) Experimental studies on the implantation of hydroxylapatite in the medullary canal of rabbits. First World Biomaterials Congress Baden near Vienna/Austria
Nizard M (1981) Knochengewebsneubildung durch Collagen-Apatit-Implantation. Habilitationsschrift, Universität Homburg
Ogino M, Okuchi F, Hench LL (1980) Compositional dependence of the formation of calcium phosphate films on bioglass. J Biomed Mater Res 14:55
Olerud S, Lorenzi G (1970) Triple fluorochrome labeling in bone formation and bone resorption. J Bone Joint Surg (Am) 52:274
Ollier L (1867) Traite experimental et clinique de la regeneration des os et de la production artificielle du tissu osseux. Masson, Paris

Orell S (1934) Studien über Knochentransplantation und Knochenneubildung. Acta Chir Scand (Suppl) 74:31
Osborn JF (1983) Hydroxylapatitkeramik. Habilitationsschrift, Universität Hamburg
Osborn, JF, Weiss T (1979) Hydroxylapatitkeramik – ein knochenähnlicher Biowerkstoff. Schweiz Monatsschr Zahnheilkd 88:1166
Osborn JF, Newseley H (1979) Dynamic aspects of the implant bone interface. Symp Enwp Soc Biomaterials, Heidelberg, März 1979
Osborn JF, Newseley H (1980) The material science of calcium phosphate ceramics. Biomaterials 1:108
Owen M (1963) Cell population kinetics of an osteogenic tissue. J Cell Biol 19:19
Owen M (1970) The origin of bone cells. Int Rev Cytol 28:213
Owen M (1980) The origin of bone cells in the postnatal organism. Arthritis Rheum 23:1073
Parfitt AM (1984) Osteoporosis: Aspects of bone remodeling and turnover. Vortrag II. Internationales Expertengespräch „Calcitonin" 13.–14. 4. 1984
Patel A (1982) Utilisation de coreaux en chirurgie orthopedique. Rev Palais Decouv 98:1
Peelen JGJ, Rejda BV, Vermeiden JPW, de Groot K (1977) Sintered tricalciumphosphate as bioceramic. Sci Ceram 9:226
Petrides PE (1979) Binde- und Stützgewebe. In: Löffler G, Petrides PE, Weiss L, Harper HA (Hrsg) Physiologische Chemie. Springer, Berlin Heidelberg New York
Plasmans CMT, Kuypers W, Slooff TJJH (1978) The effect of ethane-1-hydroxy-1, 1-diphosphonic acid (EHDP) on matrix induced ectopic bone formation. Clin Orthop 132:233
Popkirov S (1981) Entnahme autologer Knochentransplantate und gleichzeitiger osteoplastischer Ersatz des Donorknochendefektes. Zentralbl Chir 106:455
Priesack W, Bohmert H (1982) Indikationen und Anwendung lokaler Hämostyptica in der plastischen Chirurgie. In: Breddin HK, Siewert JR (Hrsg) Lokale Blutstillung. Bibliomed, Melsungen
Pucket WO (1941) The metracrylate plastics as mounting media for biological materials. Anat Rec 80:453
Puett D, Wassermann BK, Ford JD, Cuninghams LW (1973) Collagen-mediated platelet aggregation. J Clin Invest 52:2495
Rahn BA (1976) Die polychrome Sequenzmarkierung. Habilitationsschrift, Universität Freiburg
Rahn BA (1976) Die polychrome Sequenzmarkierung des Knochens. Nova Acta Leopoldina 44:249
Rahn BA, Bacellar FC, Trapp L, Perren SM (1980) Methode zur Fluoreszenz-Morphometrie des Knochenanbaus. Aktuel Traumatol 10:109
Rao WR, Boehm RF (1974) A study of sintered apatites. J Dent Res 53:1351
Rasmussen H, Bordier P (1974) The physiological and cellular basis of metabolic bone disease. Williams & Wilkins, Baltimore
Raveh J, Stich H, Rutti C (1982) Osteoplastik und Defektüberbrückung am Gesichtsschädel mit einer neuen Substanz – Biozement. Dtsch Zahnärztl Z 37:498
Ray RD, Ward AA (1952) A preliminary report on studies of basic calcium phosphate in bone replacement. Surgical Forum, Saunders, Philadelphia
Reich G (1966) Kollagen – Eine Einführung in Methoden, Ergebnisse und Probleme der Kollagenforschung. Steinkopff, Dresden
Reynolds JJ (1968) Inhibition by calcitonin of bone resorption induced in vitro by vitamin A. Proc R Soc Lond (Biol) 170:61
Rich A, Crick FHC (1961) The molecular structure of collagen. J Mol Biol 3:483
Riege W, Köhnlein HE (1978) Kollagenvlies. Chirurg 49:246
Romeis B (1968) Mikroskopische Technik. Oldenbourg, München Wien
Roofe PG, Hoecker FE, Vorhees CD (1949) A rapid bone sectioning technique. Proc Soc Exp Biol Med 72:619
Rootare HM, Powers JM, Craig RG (1977) Sintered hydroxylapatite ceramic for wear studies. J Dent Res 57:777
Rosin A, Freiberg H, Zajicek G (1963) The fabe of rat bone marrow, spleen and periosteum cultivated in vivo in the diffusion chamber, with special reforce to bone formation. Exp Cell Res 29:176
Roy DM, Linnehan SK (1974) Hydroxylapatite formed from coral skeletal carbonate by hydrothermal exchange. Nature 247:220
Rüedi TP, Bassett CAL (1967) Repair and remodeling in millipore-isolated defects in cortical bone. Acta Anat (Basel) 68:509

Runge H, Hein G, Franke J (1979) Unsere Erfahrungen mit der automatischen Bildverarbeitung von Knochenpräparaten unter besonderer Berücksichtigung der Hartschnittechnik. Beitr Orthop Traumatol 26:698
Salama R (1983) Xenogeneic bone grafting in humans. Clin Orthop 174:113
Salama R, Gazit E (1978) The antigenicity of kiel bone in the human host. J Bone Joint Surg (Br) 60:262
Saur K, Dambe LT, Schweiberer L (1978) Experimentelle Untersuchungen zum Einbau autologer Spongiosa in die Compacta des Röhrenknochens. Arch Orthop Trauma Surg 92:211
Schachtschabel DO, Blencke BA (1976) Effect of pulverized implantation materials (plastic and glass ceramic) on growth and metabolism of mammalian cell cultures. Eur Surg Res 8:71
Scharf JH (1960) Bau und Funktion des Knochens. Zentralbl Chir 17a:809
Schautz R (1962) Zur Herstellungstechnik von Konservenknochenspänen. Chirurg 33:457
Schenk R (1965) Zur histologischen Verarbeitung von unentkalkten Knochen. Acta Anat (Basel) 60:3
Schenk R (1967) Morphometrische Analyse der Umbauvorgänge in der Kompakta des Knochens. In: Weibel ER (Hrsg) Quantative Methoden in der Morphologie. Springer, Berlin Heidelberg NewYork, p 199
Schenk RK (1978) Die Histologie der primären Knochenheilung im Lichte neuer Konzeptionen über den Knochenumbau. Unfallheilkd 81:219
Schenk RK, Merz WA (1969) Histologisch-morphometrische Untersuchungen über Altersatrophie und senile Osteoporose in der Spongiosa des Beckenkamms. Dtsch Wochenschr 5:206
Schenk RK, Willenegger HR (1977) Zur Histologie der primären Knochenheilung. Modifikationen und Grenzen der Spätheilung in Abhängigkeit von der Defektgröße. Unfallheilkunde 80:155
Schenk RK, Merz WA, Müller J (1969) A quantitative histological study on bone resorption in human cancellous bone. Acta Anat (Basel) 74:44
Schilling H, Nockemann PF (1962) Histologische Betrachtungen über tierexperimentelle und klinische Erfahrungen nit einem heteroplastischen Knochenmaterial. Unfallheilkunde 65:227
Schönfeldt C, Bössmann K (1980) Eine Methacrylateinbettung zur histologischen Untersuchung entkalkter wie auch unentkalkter Präparate von Zähnen mit umgebendem Parodont. Dtsch Zahnärztl Z 35:789
Schönmayr R, Schepelmann F (1982) Besonderheiten der Blutstillung bei Eingriffen am zentralen Nervensystem. In: Breddin HK, Siewert JR (Hrsg) Lokale Blutstillung. Bibliomed, Melsungen
Schramm W (1970) Klinische und experimentelle Untersuchungen über die Transplantation autoplastischer Spongiosa. Hefte Unfallheilkunde 104. Springer, Berlin Heidelberg New York
Schumacher S (1934) Grundriß der Histologie des Menschen. Springer, Wien
Schweiberer L (1970) Experimentelle Untersuchungen von Knochentransplantaten mit unveränderter und mit denaturierter Knochengrundsubstanz. Hefte Unfallheilkunde 103. Springer, Berlin Heidelberg NewYork
Schweiberer L (1976) Theoretisch experimentelle Grundlagen der autologen Spongiosatransplantation im Infekt. Hefte Unfallheilkunde 79:151. Springer, Berlin Heidelberg NewYork
Schweiberer L, Brenneisen R, Dambe LT, Eitel F, Zwank L (1981) Derzeitiger Stand der auto-, hetero- und homoplastischen Knochentransplantation. In: Cotta H, Martini AK (Hrsg) Implantate und Transplantate in der Plastischen und Wiederherstellungschirurgie. Springer, Berlin Heidelberg NewYork, S 115
Scott BL (1967) Thymidine ^{3}H electron microscope radioautography of osteogenic cells in the fetal rat. J Cell Bio 35:115
Segmüller G (1967) Spongiosaregeneration in der Milliporekammer. Helv Chir Acta 34:5
Senn N (1889) On the healing of aseptic bone cavities by implantation of antiseptic decalcified bone. Am J Med Sci 98:219
Shima T, Keller JT, Alriva MM, Mayfield FH, Dunsker SB (1979) Anterior cervical discectomy and interbody fusion. J Neurosurg 51:533
Shoshan S, Gross J (1974) Biosynthesis and metabolism of collagen and its role in tissue repair processes. Isr Med Sci 10:537
Siebert J, Laible B, Konold P, Pannike A, Schröder R (1976) Automatische quantitative Auswertung von Knochenbiopsien. Vergleichende Untersuchungen verschiedener Färbemethoden und Microradiographien. Unfallchirurgie 2:76
Skinner HCW, Kittelberger JS, Beebe RA (1975) Thermal instability in synthetic hydroxyapatites. J Phys Chem 79:2017
Smith JW (1968) Molecular pattern in native collagen. Nature 219:157

Snyder AJ, Levin MP (1979) Osteogenic potential of ceramic implants placed into peridontal defects in humans (Abstracts). IADR 57th General Session New Orleans, p 1095
Spängler HP, Braun F, Holle J, Moritz E, Wolner E (1976) Die lokale Anwendung von Fibrin und Kollagen zur Blutstillung in der Herzchirurgie. Wien Med Wochenschr 7:86
Spence KF, Sell KW, Brown RH (1969) Solitary bone cyst: Treatment with freeze-dried cancellous bone allograft. J Bone Joint Surg (Am) 51:87
Spence KF, Bright RW, Fitzgerald SP, Sell KW (1976) Solitary unicameral bone cyst: Treatment with freezedried crushed cortical bone allograft. J Bone Joint Surg (Am) 58:636
Springorum HW (1980) Tierexperimentelle Untersuchungen der Knochenregeneration nach Kollagenimplantation in standardisierten Knochendefekten an der Ratte, am Kaninchen, an wachsenden und ausgewachsenen Hunden. Habilitationsschrift, Universität Heidelberg
Springorum HW, Adler CP, Jäger W, Ober E (1977) Tierexperimentelle Untersuchung der Knochenregeneration am standardisierten Tibiadefekt des Kaninchens nach Implantation von Kollagenvlies im Vergleich zur autologen und homologen Spongiosaplastik. Z Orthop 115:686
Steffen C, Ludwig H, Thumb N, Frank O, Eberl R, Tausch F (1973) Nachweis von Antikörpern mit verschiedener Kollagenspezifität bei progressiv chronischer Polyarthritis und Vergleich vom Humankollagen und Kalbskollagen als Testantigen. Klin Wochenschr 51:222
Steinmann B, Gitzelmann R (1984) Das Kollagen im Bindegewebe: Vom Leim zur Molekularstruktur. Ortopädie 13:3
Stemberger A, Fritsche HM, Primbs P, Blümel G (1978) Fibrinogenkonzentrate und Kollagenschwämme zur Gewebeklebung. Med Welt 29:721
Stockamp C (1982) Urologie. In: Breddin HK, Siewert JR (Hrsg) Lokale Blutstillung. Bibliomed, Melsungen
Strates B, Neuman WF (1958) On the mechanisms of calcification. Proc Soc Exp Biol Med 97:688
Stryer L (1979) Biochemie. Vieweg, Braunschweig
Tannenbaum PJ, Schraer H, Posner AS (1974) Crystalline changes in avian related on the reproductive cycle. Calcif Tissue Res 14:83
Taylor GJ, Miller GDH, Ham FJ (1975) The free vascularized bone graft. Plast Reconstr Surg 55:533
Teitelbaum SL, Bates M (1980) Relationship of static and kinetic histomorphometric features of bone. Clin Orthop 146:239
Termine JD (1972) Mineral chemistry and skeletal biology. Clin Orthop 85:207
Thielemann FW, Veihelmann D, Schmidt K (1978) Die Induktion der Knochenneubildung nach Transplantation. Arch Orthop Trauma Surg 91:3
Thielemann FW, Veihelmann D, Schmidt K (1979) Osteogenetische Wirkung von Knochenmatrix und Knochengelatine. Hefte Unfallheilkd 148:241
Thielemann FW, Späth G, Veihelmann D, Schmidt K (1982a) Osteoinduction, part 1. Arch Orthop Trauma Surg 99:217
Thielemann FW, Späth G, Veihelmann D, Schmidt K (1982b) Osteoinduction. Arch Orthop Trauma Surg 100:73
Tomford WW, Doppelt SH, Mankin HJ, Friedlaender GE (1983) 1983 Bone bank procedures. Clin Orthop 174:15
Tuli SM, Singh AD (1978) The osteoinductive property of decalcified bone matrix. J Bone Joint Surg (Br) 60:116
Urist MR (1965) Bone: Formation by autoinduction. Science 150:893
Urist MR, Dowell TA (1968) The inductive substratum for osteogenesis in pellets of particular bone matrix. Clin Orthop 61:61
Urist MR, Mikulski A, Boyd SD (1975) A chemosterilized antigen-extracted autodigested alloimplant for bone banks. Arch Surg 110:416
Urist MR, Lietze A, Dawson E (1984) β-tricalcium phosphate delivery system for bone morphogenetic protein. Clin Orthop 187:277
Vaughan J (1975) The physiology of bone. Clarendon, Oxford
Veihelmann D, Thielemann F (1976) Bestimmungsmethode für konservierungsbedingte Wertigkeitseinbuße bei Knochentransplantaten. Hefte Unfallheilkd 79:305
de Vernejoul MC, Kuntz D, Miravet L, Goutallier D, Ryckewaert A (1981) Bone histomorphometric reproducibility in normal patients. Calcif Tissue Int 33:369
Vistness LM, Goodwin DA, Tenery JH, Ksauder GA, Gruber RP (1974) Control of cap illary bleeding by topical application of microcrystalline collagen. Surgery 76:291

Wagner W, Tetsch P, Ackermann KL, Böhmer U, Dahl H (1981) Tierexperimentelle Untersuchungen zur Knochenregeneration genormter Defekte nach der Implantation einer Trikalziumphosphatkeramik. Dtsch Zahnärztl Z 36:82
Watson RF, Rothbard S, Vanamel P (1954) The antigenicity of rat collagen. J Exp Med 99:535
Weber M (1985) Tierexperimentelle Untersuchungen zur Knochenregeneration mit gereinigtem, xenogenem Faserkollagen und Apatitpulver. Inauguraldissertation, Universität Homburg
Weiland AJ, Moore JR, Daniel RK (1983) Vascularized bone autografts: Experience with 41 cases. Clin Orthop 174:87
Westen H, Mück KF, Post L (1981) Enzyme histochemistry on bone marrow sections after embedding in methacrylate at low temperature. Histochemistry 70:95
Willenegger H, Perren SM, Schenk R (1971) Primäre und sekundäre Knochenbruchheilung. Chirurg 6:241
Wuppermann T, Hörmann H (1974) Biochemische Prozesse bei der Auslösung der Blutgerinnung durch Kollagen. Klin Wochenschr 52:409
Young RW (1962) Regional differences in cell generation time in growing rat tibial. Exp Cell Res 26:562
Young RW (1963) Nucleid acids, protein synthesis and bone. Clin Orthop 26:147
Young RW (1975) Biological apatite vs hydroxylapatite at the atomic level. Clin Orthop 113:249

Subject Index

J. Wolff

The Law of Bone Remodelling

Translated from the German by P. Maquet, R. Furlong

1986. 95 figures. XII, 126 pages.
ISBN 3-540-16281-X

Julius Wolff's book is mentioned in about every work dealing with bone structure. His name is familiar to every anatomist and orthopaedic surgeon. Very few, however, have actually read his book, written in the flowery scientific German of the turn of the century. A translation into English was thus needed to make the work available to a larger audience interested in the problems of bone structure.

Julius Wolff, studying thin slices of bone at the end of the last century, observed the pattern formed by the cancellous trabeculae and continuing into the cortices. He noticed changes in this pattern after malunited fractures or in otherwise deformed bones and attributed these modifications to the change in mechanical stressing which resulted from the bone deformation. He attempted to relate the patterns he observed in the trajectories of compressive and tensile stresses to the then recent theories of Culmann on resistance of materials and elasticity. He thereby started a hundred-year discussion about the trajectorial structure of bone which was only concluded in 1973 by Pauwels. This book is the basis on which different theses were elaborated by the greatest anatomists of the last hundred years.

Springer Verlag
Berlin Heidelberg
New York London
Paris Tokyo

Springer

GPSR Compliance

The European Union's (EU) General Product Safety Regulation (GPSR) is a set of rules that requires consumer products to be safe and our obligations to ensure this.

If you have any concerns about our products, you can contact us on ProductSafety@springernature.com

In case Publisher is established outside the EU, the EU authorized representative is:

Springer Nature Customer Service Center GmbH
Europaplatz 3
69115 Heidelberg, Germany

Batch number: 10704763

Printed by Printforce, the Netherlands